ANNA GEARY

Anna's Game Plan

Conquer Your Hang-ups,
Unlock Your Confidence and
Find Your Purpose

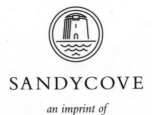

SANDYCOVE

an imprint of

PENGUIN BOOKS

SANDYCOVE

UK | USA | Canada | Ireland | Australia
India | New Zealand | South Africa

Sandycove is part of the Penguin Random House group of companies
whose addresses can be found at global.penguinrandomhouse.com.

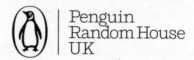

First published 2024

001

Copyright © Anna Geary, 2024

The moral right of the author has been asserted

Set in 13.6/16.2pt Adobe Garamond Pro
Typeset by Jouve (UK), Milton Keynes
Printed and bound in Great Britain by Clays Ltd, Elcograf S.p.A.

The authorized representative in the EEA is Penguin Random House Ireland,
Morrison Chambers, 32 Nassau Street, Dublin D02 YH68

A CIP catalogue record for this book is available from the British Library

ISBN: 978–1–844–88643–2

www.greenpenguin.co.uk

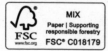

Anna's Game Plan

For Ronan.

Dream your dreams, chase them hard
and never be afraid to be yourself
while pursuing them.

'The only person you are destined to become
is the person you decide to be'
– Ralph Waldo Emerson

Contents

Introduction: Game Plan for Life

'Your playing small does not serve the world. There's
nothing enlightened about shrinking so that other
people won't feel insecure around you'
– Marianne Williamson, *A Return to Love*

Given the busy nature of our daily lives, with all the stresses
and demands placed upon us, it's only natural that we some-
times lose sight of who we are or what we want out of our
lives. We can all live on autopilot mode, going through the
motions but not really engaging fully with ourselves. We tell
ourselves that tomorrow, next week, next month, next year
will be different, and yet we find ourselves on the same inter-
minable merry-go-round, unable or unwilling to get off.

I am no stranger to this. Days sometimes fly past in a haze
of busyness, where I'm constantly on the go. And don't get me
wrong, I enjoy being busy: it gives me a sense of purpose. But
sometimes you need to sit down and take stock, think about
what will make you happy in both the short- and long-term.

For me, the idea for this book has been swirling around my
head for some time. There's nothing I love more than spend-
ing a quiet hour browsing in a bookshop. I love the sense of

peace and calm that envelops me as I scan the bookshelves, seeking inspiration, motivation, solace and encouragement. There's nothing better than a book to help you disconnect from real life for a while. Immersing yourself in the words and worlds of others is balm for the soul. That is the true power of a book.

I passionately wanted to write this book, but I kept putting it off. I have asked myself so many times, why did I resist writing it? Allowing myself the time to sit and absorb myself fully in the writing process was one practical reason. But, being honest, there were much more fundamental reasons, and I guess you could say time was just a convenient excuse. In reality, it was the fear of judgement from others – I could almost hear the 'Who does she think she is?' remarks in my head. It was the fear of unrealistic expectations, mine more so than anyone else's. And it was because of doubt – doubting the capabilities that, deep down, I felt I possessed. And more than all of these, I worried whether I was enough.

Something I have learned over the course of my career and life experience to date is that many of us struggle with this feeling – the feeling of not being, not having, not doing enough.

What even is *enough*? I don't earn *enough* money. I can't lose *enough* weight. I don't go out *enough*. I haven't achieved *enough* status in my job. I haven't had *enough* success in my life.

How do you decide what *enough* is? Or does someone else decide it for you? Is it others' barometer of *enough* that you live by? We convince ourselves that if we could just get to

2

the next thing – to lose two stone, to get promoted, to buy a bigger house, to afford a designer bag – our lives would be so much better, and then we would be happy. As you read this book, I want to help you to define what *enough* means to you, in your life, so that you can learn to be happy right now.

The power of saying yes

I'm sure I'm not the only one who can say that there have been times in my life when I questioned whether I was good enough or if I was doing enough. Be it studying for exams, training for sports teams, preparing for radio or TV shows, and even in personal relationships. That negative voice in my head always had the power to drown out the reassuring voice.

The power of that negative internal voice means that we can often be too terrified to try. There's a crippling fear of stepping outside of our comfort zones in case something doesn't work out. But what if it *does* work out? *What if* on the other side of that comfort zone are opportunities you deserve to experience?

All you need do is to move out of your own way and be willing to say yes. Yes, you are enough, and yes, you can do it.

I wrote this book for that very reason. To say yes to an opportunity, to see what was on the other side of my comfort zone, because – and believe me when I say this – I have never been so far outside my comfort zone as I have been during this writing process. I am not an expert, and I can only offer the insights I've learned over the course of my journey, only share with you my own lived experience.

I've played with the Cork Senior camogie team for twelve years.

I've captained the team to All-Ireland success.

I've won All-Stars awards and have amassed over twenty All-Ireland medals during my sporting career.

I have been a coach and mentor on the popular RTÉ TV show *Ireland's Fittest Family* for almost a decade (and won it three times, but who's counting?!).

I have presented TV and radio shows. I have stood on stages and spoken to thousands of people across the country in my career as an executive and performance coach.

I have been a finalist on *Dancing with the Stars* and was the 2014 Cork Rose of Tralee.

And yet, somehow, this book has given me more sleepless nights and a deeper feeling of nervous energy than anything else I've ever done. I've poured myself into this book at a time of constant change in my life. Enduring a global pandemic, supporting a sick parent, grieving a parent, going through my first pregnancy. I've experienced it all while writing this book.

But I did it, I faced my fears, I drowned out my inner critic, I worked to the best of my abilities, and I persevered. I found that there is power in the discomfort too, and strength in the vulnerability that it has unearthed within me.

Figuring out what you think about you

In this book, I want to help you reconnect. To reconnect with your whole self, with your everyday reality and with your dreams. I want to help you to reconnect to what you really want to achieve from life, instead of what you think you might want, or who you think you should be. You might have to shed some long-established habits, and change the way you view yourself, but in doing so, you can unlock the true version of yourself, a version of you that is ready to live life to the full.

Throughout the writing process, I often felt like I was talking directly to both my younger self and to my present self. It enabled me to remind myself that I am capable, determined and competitive, full of passion and enthusiasm. It also allowed me to acknowledge that I tend to overanalyse situations, be excessively self-critical and struggle with self-confidence. It allowed me to reflect on my career and understand that it enabled me to do what I love best, which is working with other people.

I get immense energy and joy in helping others to improve and develop their personal relationships with themselves through the myriad of roles I have found myself in: coach, broadcaster, speaker, captain and teammate. I'm hoping that this book might help you unlock some fundamental truths about yourself in the way that it has helped me. If my words can act as a support to you then it was worth every minute, even the tearful ones.

Over the past few years, I have focused and worked on

the relationship I have with myself – with both my mind and my body – and it's this knowledge I have gained that I want to share with you, focusing on the concepts of Acceptance, Purpose, Consistency, Challenge and Kindness. In exploring aspects of each of these topics, I'm hoping that you will gain the confidence to say yes to opportunities, yes to challenges – yes to life.

How many of us say no to opportunities, not because we don't want to explore them but because we don't have the confidence to say yes, or we worry about what others will think? This book is for anyone who wants and needs to back themselves more. It's time to care less about what others think about you and focus more on what YOU think about you.

We constantly demand so much of ourselves. We give ourselves such a hard time for stumbling, for stalling, for being uncertain or indecisive and for coming up short. The destructive voice in our heads can intensify in all these situations:

Why did you do that?

What is wrong with you?

I can't believe you did that.

But . . . in these moments are the lessons, the learnings and the growth that can elevate us to a higher level of experiencing life. These are the stories of resilience and perseverance that we will come back to again and again when talking to our kids and grandkids. Embrace and celebrate these stories too. Because it takes guts to try.

Being involved in high-level sport has afforded me opportunities to work on my mindset: to challenge my thinking, to reflect on my habits and to re-evaluate my priorities along the way. In the lead-up to my first Senior Club All-Ireland Semi-Final back in spring 2013, we had a final team meeting that I will always remember. We were going into the game as underdogs, facing the current All-Ireland Champions on their home turf. We had never reached that far in the competition before, so it was new territory for us. We were full of doubt and insecurity. Were we enough?

Two questions were put to us in the meeting:

'Are you willing?'

'Are you able?'

These are questions I have come back to again and again since then. I have challenged myself with these questions throughout different moments in my life, whether it be tough gym sessions, coping with grief, demanding job interviews, struggles with body image, and everything in between.

Am I willing?

Am I able?

During the times in life when you are faced with difficult challenges, hard decisions and tricky moments, my hope for you after reading this book is that you will have the tools, techniques and tips to help you feel *willing* and *able* to cope with anything that life throws at you.

We all need to be reminded in our lives that we can do tough things.

YOU CAN DO TOUGH THINGS!

A game plan for your future

I want to enable and empower you to drive forward, towards creating the life YOU want to live. So, whatever the reasons are that brought you to this book, you are here. Now, it's time to get excited about what's to come.

Learn to love and **accept** you for who you are and have confidence in your abilities – because you are capable of great things.

Learn to identify your **purpose**, set goals and keep motivated to achieve what you want out of your life.

Learn to embrace **consistency** in your life – discover how to show up for yourself and for others.

Learn to reframe **challenges** as opportunities. Stepping outside your comfort zone, confronting your fears and focusing on progress can be genuinely life-changing.

Learn to demonstrate **kindness** in daily life. Showing compassion to both yourself and others can unlock an unparalleled sense of happiness and contentment.

Together, let's go for it, create your game plan and put it into action.

Record your thoughts and progress

This book is called *Anna's Game Plan,* but my ambition is that as you read it you will feel empowered to come up with your own personal game plan that is a fit for your life.

On a practical note, you will find it useful to have a notebook or journal handy to jot down your ideas and reflections and to do the exercises I've shared. There are also some blank pages at the end of each part of the book where you can make notes and record your own takeaway tactics.

As well as being a source of encouragement today, I hope you can use this book as an ongoing resource, a tool you'll continue to use to review and revise your game plan as things change in life – because the one thing we all know is that nothing stays the same!

PART ONE

Game Plan for Acceptance

1. The liberating power of self-acceptance

'You are allowed to be both a masterpiece
and a work in progress, simultaneously'
– Sophia Bush

Self-acceptance isn't easy. It's something I have struggled with over the years. But by going through this struggle, I have learned that accepting my whole self – the good and the bad – can be truly liberating. It allows for a level of contentment in my life that I might not have if I was constantly criticizing myself. And don't get me wrong, I'm not immune to negative thoughts snaking their way into my mind, but I've learned ways of reframing this negative narrative into a positive.

Learning to accept yourself – your body, your personality, your flaws, your strengths, the inner essence of who you are as a person – is a journey. In this section of the book, I'll share with you some of my experiences with self-acceptance, and some tricks and tips I've learned along the way.

When I was younger, my grandmother always used to say to me 'what people think about you is none of your business'.

And now, whenever I feel anxious in some way about how I might be perceived, I always think of this saying. You cannot control how you are perceived by other people. They will make up their minds about who you are as a person, whether it's accurate or not. But if you don't know who you are, you can be shaken by the perceptions that others have of you. Ultimately, you can only control how you see yourself. And you can learn to be your biggest cheerleader.

Over the years, as a high-level sportsperson, media broadcaster and coach, I've had to develop coping mechanisms to deal with negativity – negativity that I have felt about myself and negativity I have received from other people. I have been met with negative comments about the way I speak, about my personality and about my appearance. I have had to learn how to deal with the level of negativity directed at me or else I wouldn't be able to survive in this industry. But many of us deal with a similar kind of challenge daily, both professionally and personally – not to mention with the pervasiveness of social media in our lives. We tend to care more about what others think about us than what we think about ourselves.

Your critics are not your best advisors

A few years ago, I was invited to join *The Sunday Game* panel on RTÉ as a hurling analyst. I had been involved in the camogie coverage as an analyst since 2015 but being asked to join and talk about the men's game was brilliant, if a little daunting. Why? It wasn't because I felt that I wouldn't have anything to contribute. I have played in countless All-Ireland Finals. I understand the game of hurling, and back my own opinions around it. However, I was acutely aware of an attitude that exists among a certain cohort of people that whenever they see a woman talking about men's sport, they instantly dismiss her and refer to her as the 'token woman'.

It was an honour to be asked, so I said yes, and on my first day I stood shoulder to shoulder with two former hurling stars. I was nervous but I enjoyed the panel discussion. Did I feel the pressure? Absolutely. But as American tennis legend Billie Jean King once said, 'pressure is a privilege', so I tried to embrace it.

I gave my opinion, commented on the match from my perspective, and generally got involved in the conversation. My opinions were listened to by the other analysts and, overall, I was happy when we came off-air. It wasn't until afterwards that I became aware of the negative criticism from some people online. They wrote that I took over the panel. I interrupted the men too much, I said too much. I was taken aback because I didn't feel that this was a true reflection of the panel discussion. It seemed to me that, on the playing field, people applauded my determination and self-assuredness, but off the field those traits were expected to disappear. I had to turn off that fire and that passion.

I was simply doing my job, but I took note of what they said and I decided to hold back a bit the next time. Looking back now, I was compromising myself to be more pleasing to others – whoever they were – and more self-contained. It felt wrong to sit nodding during a conversation about a sport

I had played my whole life, a sport I had reached the top of my game in more than once. I consciously listened more than I contributed. Afterwards, I was again criticized online. This time it was for my facial expressions. My attentiveness and concentration were mistaken for scowling, while I was also accused of not saying enough. I couldn't win.

In the end, I decided to ignore those other voices. I would listen to my own voice and the voices of my support circle. A friend of mine said something that hit home: 'If you wouldn't take their advice, why would you listen to their criticism?' Read that quote again because it might resonate with you too. We call these types of people keyboard warriors, but there is nothing warrior-like about what they do. Instead, we should call them keyboard cowards, hiding behind a screen, pointing out the mistakes and faults of others. It's far easier to do that than to embrace the pressure that comes with trying something yourself.

I am the same person both on and off the field, whether it's playing camogie, coaching on *Ireland's Fittest Family*, speaking to corporate groups, or if you meet me on the street. My persona, my passion, my competitiveness, my work ethic, my drive . . . it's evident. Why should I be made to feel I have to turn it off? I only know how to be me. And so I've decided that's who I am going to be.

Why should any one of us need to be *less* because someone thinks we are too much? It says more about them than it does about ourselves. I'm determined and ambitious. I have learned to embrace these qualities. I have accepted that they make me who I am.

Why are we waiting for external validation to come from others? Do you let others decide if you are to be accepted? Think about the ways you might be letting that happen in your life. Instead, you need to strive for self-acceptance. This will help to build self-confidence and give you greater freedom, so that *you* can decide the best course of action for your life.

2. The acceptance mindset

'You can be the ripest, juiciest peach in the world,
but still meet someone who hates peaches'
– Dita Von Teese

Looking outwards for acceptance is impossible: there will
always be someone who you don't gel with; there will always
be people, for whatever reason, who just don't like you. But
you can like you – your relationship with yourself is the foun-
dation for everything. It affects all that you do, how you pre-
sent yourself, your relationships with other people, your job,
everything. So, it's important to check on that foundation
regularly, and to make sure you maintain it.

Have you ever seen a bricklayer at work? They make it
look so easy, don't they? But we know that they are skilled in
their craft. They've spent years learning the specific process
that they need to follow. You would never expect to build a
house in a day. We know houses are built on land that has
been surveyed and prepared, before solid foundations can
be placed, before the bricks can be laid. If you were build-
ing anything, you would take time, effort and care with it to
make sure it would last, to make sure it wouldn't fall down

or fall apart. Think of your life, and your journey through it, as a self-build. Give yourself time, care and love, and you will build a good foundation, and then build up brick by brick until you are able to weather the storm of outside critique and opinion.

Loving yourself and being confident in your capabilities and who you are doesn't mean that you live without fear, doubt, worries or regrets. There is no end point, no final destination on this journey – it involves constant practice. Getting into this mindset can be difficult, but not impossible, and I want to share with you a few exercises and tips that I've found helpful, and which might help you too.

Practise compassion

'If you want others to be happy, practise compassion.
If you want to be happy, practise compassion'
– Dalai Lama

Often, we are our own worst enemies, our own harshest crit-ics. I think I can safely say that I'm not the only one who has a little voice ringing through my head at times, telling me I'm not good enough, berating me for my faults, ques-tioning my actions. The central theory of self-compassion is accepting that we are all imperfect, we all make mistakes at times, we all have flaws – so instead of relentlessly criticiz-ing ourselves, we embrace ourselves for who we truly are as people. Self-compassion is recognizing that life is a shared experience – we all go through challenging times, and we all fail at times. It is not a unique state of being. When we practise self-compassion, we will find that we have an increased personal drive to make positive changes in our lives.

Empowering yourself

You will start to become an unshakeable force within your own life when you work on things that no one can take away from you.

Your self-compassion, your self-belief, your self-worth. They all start with the inner self. No outside influences necessary.

When I look back at my extraordinary time on *Dancing with the Stars*, I can't believe that I almost turned it down. I have always been a girl who loved to dance – from ill-advised *Riverdance*-esque leaps around my childhood kitchen to pretending to be a Spice Girl with my friends (I was always Sporty Spice – shocker, I know!). Dancing made me feel happy and free. But the offer really threw me.

At the time, I was at the beginning of regenerating my professional life, in a period of transition and trying to work out a new identity. I had been a sportsperson for so long, 'Anna Geary, the Cork camogie player', but now that I was retired and had started to dip my toe into media broadcasting,

I still hadn't quite figured out who I was. The show was offering me an opportunity to explore a different side of myself away from my career in sports, a new one in broadcasting, and it offered me exactly what I needed at exactly the right time. So why was I so hesitant?

The truth was that I was terrified of being judged, and of what people would say about me. Would people think I had notions about myself for appearing on a show filled with well-known Irish stars and media personalities when I was just a camogie player from a rural village in North Cork? And this is before I had even contemplated what they would say about my looks, my body and the small matter of my dancing ability.

It took all my inner resolve to force myself out of my comfort zone to say yes. I had to ignore my self-critical, vulnerable side and reframe my negative thoughts. I had to practise self-compassion and identify what I really wanted. I asked myself those two questions: *Am I willing? Am I able?* I could do it, and I would do it. I would treat myself with the compassion I deserved and would support and encourage myself. I knew that being on this show could make me happy. I love dancing, I love a challenge, and it was an exciting opportunity.

Sometimes we lose sight of who we really are and what we really want because we are too concerned about being judged or failing. And at times over the seventeen weeks, I was faced with tough challenges, emotionally, mentally and physically. But what I got back in terms of enjoyment, friendships and incredible memories was worth it all. I'm glad I silenced the inner negative critic by exercising self-compassion, and it enabled me to move forward in my career in such a positive way.

Sometimes we just need to say yes to opportunities and then we can figure everything else out afterwards. But once you say no, you have cut yourself off from those new possibilities.

Banish negative self-talk

'A negative mind will never give you a positive life'
– Buddha

One thing that helped me to make this positive decision to do *Dancing with the Stars* was to separate myself from what I perceived to be the judgement of others, and to listen to my inner voice and the self-talk I engaged with every day. Often our self-talk can be negative – 'Why didn't I do this?' if you made a decision that didn't work out, or 'I'm worthless because I got that wrong' if you made a mistake at work. Negative self-talk can be so damaging. It can limit your ability to believe in yourself and your talents, and it might hinder your attempts to reach your full potential in life.

Well then, how do we limit our negative self-talk? The answer is compassion: you find an inner conversation that still describes the same reality, but in a much more compassionate way. So instead of saying 'What if I completely mess up and make a show of myself on national TV?' I chose to reframe it to 'What if I have the best experience, learn a new skill and it sets me on a new career path?'

This way of compassionate thinking is empowering. It allows you to do things that you need to do to progress, to feel a sense of achievement and contentment in life. They don't need to be life-changing decisions, but this can help with the many little decisions you have to make in everyday life.

Be aware of your mindset triggers, reaction and inner voice. Notice when you are saying to yourself:

'I can't do this.'

'I've made a mistake and people will think I can't do my job.'

'My co-worker is more efficient than me.'

Stop for a moment. Consciously choose a different way of thinking about a situation:

'How can I learn to do this?'

'How can I learn from my mistake?'

'What can I learn from her?'

By embracing a more positive mindset you will actively seek ways to improve, to look more positively on a situation and be more likely to perform better.

Nightly reflection

Take a few minutes at the end of the day to reflect on your self-talk. You can use a journal if this helps. Write down any self-judgements you made to yourself during the day.

When you are looking over them, ask yourself if they are true or critical statements. Ask yourself if you could rephrase them in a more compassionate way. For example, instead of berating yourself for the things you didn't get done that day, praise yourself for the things you *did* achieve.

Some quick tips on limiting negative self-talk:

- **Say it out loud** – if you find you're engaging in negative self-talk, say it out loud. Sometimes it helps us realize how ridiculous it actually sounds, and it can help to stop that line of negativity quickly.
- **Shift your perspective** – when you're criticizing yourself for some decision or a mistake you made, shift your perspective. Ask yourself if it will matter in a week, six months, a year's time.
- **Try to remember that your thoughts and feelings often aren't reflective of reality** – we are all influenced by our own biases and moods, and sometimes they paint a skewed reality. Try to focus on what's really happening and insert some objectivity into your thoughts.

Talk to yourself as you would a loved one

Acknowledge what you are saying and ask yourself:
'If I was saying these exact words to a loved one,
how would they react?'

Speak to yourself as you would to a close loved one.
If they were going through the same experience that
you are going through, what would you say to them?
Would you be mean and unkind to them? No. So,
please stop being mean to yourself.

Even if it was a situation where they did something
wrong, it is likely that you would show them support
and compassion.

We are all capable of saying or doing the wrong
thing, or making a wrong decision, and it is
important to recognize the wrong, but not to be
self-punitive, to show the same compassion to
yourself that you would extend to a friend or family
member.

Breaking the negative thought loop

'The happiness of your life depends
upon the quality of your thoughts'
— Marcus Aurelius

One of my biggest everyday struggles is the fear of getting
something wrong in a relationship – either personal or busi-
ness, crucial or minor. I hate the idea of upsetting other people
because I value connection and my reputation so highly. I
reread an email a dozen times before I send it in case I've
said something 'wrong', and when someone doesn't reply to
me quickly, I get myself caught up in an imaginary scenario
where I've mortally offended them.

The average person has around 6,200 thoughts in a
single day, and over 90 per cent of these thoughts are repeti-
tive.* If we are constantly thinking negative thoughts about
ourselves, or worrying about a specific situation or problem,
it is repeated over and over again, amplifying itself each time
we think about it.

With every negative, self-punishing thought, we condition
a belief system in our subconscious mind to become stronger
and stronger, and our feelings and actions will result from that
conditioned response. Our beliefs and experiences can have an
impact on the types of thoughts we have daily – and because

---

* Tseng, J., and Poppenk, J., 'Brain meta-state transitions demarcate thoughts
across task contexts exposing the mental noise of trait neuroticism', *Nature
Communications* 11, 3480 (2020). https://doi.org/10.1038/s41467-020-17255-9

our thoughts, emotions and behaviours are inextricably linked to these, they have an impact on how we think and act.

Having negative thoughts is a universal experience, and we all know that negative thoughts are not helpful for us. They can impact our decisions, our behaviours and our motivation in a destructive way. But can we actively do something to change the pattern? First, we need to be able to identify our negative thought patterns before we can learn how to break the pattern. I've listed some common negative thought patterns below – see how many you recognize in yourself.

- **All-or-nothing thinking** – this is when you tend to view yourself as either a complete success or a complete failure in every situation. There is no middle ground.
- **Jumping to conclusions** – this distortion involves making assumptions about what others are thinking or making negative assumptions about how events will turn out.
- **Catastrophizing** – this is characterized by assuming that the worst possible outcome will happen without considering more likely and realistic possibilities.
- **Overgeneralization** – this is a tendency to apply what happened in one experience to all future experiences. This can make negative experiences seem unavoidable and contribute to feelings of anxiety.

- **Labelling** – this occurs when, or if, you label yourself in a negative way, and it affects how you feel about yourself. For example, if you label yourself as 'bad at running', you will often feel negative about any activities that involve running.
- **'Should' statements** – thinking marked by 'should' statements contributes to a negative perspective, leading you to think only in terms of what you 'should' be doing. These statements often tend to be unrealistic and cause you to feel defeated and pessimistic about your ability to succeed.
- **Emotional reasoning** – this is the assumption that something is true based on your emotional response to it. For example, if you are feeling nervous, emotional reasoning might lead you to think that you must be in danger. This can increase negative feelings and increase your anxiety levels.
- **Personalization and blame** – this thought pattern is when you take things personally, even when they are not personal. It often leads to you blaming yourself for something you have no control over.

As you can see, all these thinking patterns vary in slightly different ways, but they all involve distortion of reality and irrational ways of looking at situations and people.

In my earlier days playing with Cork, there would be occasions when I couldn't make it to training and would have to let my manager know. Those texts were so tough for me to send because I genuinely got myself into this crazy negative spin where I would imagine my manager reading the text, shaking his head and talking to the management team about me.

It was made worse if he didn't respond for a while. I would conjure up a multitude of reasons to explain why he wasn't texting me back. Maybe he felt that I wasn't committed to the team and this would give him the perfect excuse to drop me? I would go through all the emotions as if I was being dropped. Looking back now, it was crazy – I can see how absurd it was because I always had a legitimate excuse for missing training that was totally reasonable.

The story always ended the same way, with a thumbs-up from my manager or a response saying, 'No bother, see you next week,' and I would be flooded with the relief of knowing that I was still on the team. It would be the same if I had to cancel on someone, or say no to a job, or anything negative at all. I would overthink it. Then I learned about a theory called the *negative thought loop*.

A thought is merely a thought

The negative thought loop occurs when our mind latches on to something and keeps mulling it over and over without any real benefit. It could be something as simple as a comment online or an offhand response from a friend, and it starts to play on a loop in your head, and each time it loops, the reaction of stress kicks in again. You spend the day in turmoil, only to go online later and see that the person has replied and apologized for being crabby, explaining it had

29

nothing to do with you, or your friend has texted to see if you want to meet for a drink because she's had a bad day. So, you've wasted the entire day analysing your friendship, or thinking terrible things about yourself for no reason. You catastrophized.

The issue is that your brain can't tell what's real and what's just you being irrational, so it acts as though the situation is actually happening and responds accordingly. Over and over again, all day. Negative thought loops love company too, so your thoughts could spiral and suddenly you begin to tell yourself that not only will everyone hate you but you will probably never amount to anything and you're a failure and that's just how it is, so you may as well never leave the house again.

Tied in with the concept of the negative thought loop is *negativity bias*. Negativity bias can cause our emotional response to negative situations or experiences to feel amplified compared with similar positive experiences. For example, ten people can pay you a nice compliment about your outfit, but if one person remarks in a negative way, that's the one you tend to dwell on. The reason being is that we are naturally inclined to internalize negative experiences or comments more deeply due to evolution.

Negativity bias has been built into our brains over millions of years, as people had to pay attention to dangerous and negative threats in the world because it was literally a matter of life or death. It makes sense when you think of people having to survive in the wild millions of years ago, having to detect and avoid danger, but it's a bit harder to understand when it comes to hearing or seeing negative or demeaning comments about ourself. The brain doesn't know the difference between actual threats and perceived threats, so although our environments have changed and we are no longer hiding from predators, our brains are still hard-wired with preservation and safety in mind. When our brain perceives a threat, it responds in the same way. We can't do anything about that process – it is there to help us stay alive, after all – but we can know it, recognize it and figure out pathways around it.

When you are plagued with negative thoughts, just think of this scenario. Remember when we were children and we used to enjoy lying on the grass and watching the clouds? We would observe that they all came in different sizes. Some hung around longer than others, some morphed into different shapes, but inevitably they all moved on. Thoughts are like clouds: it's okay to acknowledge them, because they are there, but it's also okay to let them float on by. Thoughts are not always based on fact. At the end of the day, a thought is just a thought, it's the power you give it that makes it affect you.

Tips to break a negative thought loop:

- **Write it down** – by writing down what you are thinking it engages the logical side of your brain rather than the imaginative part of your brain, which can blow things out of proportion or dramatize a situation. Now examine the thought objectively. Fact-check it. Is this *actually* what is happening right now?

- **Distraction** – this can be a way to take your focus off the negative thinking, therefore breaking the cycle, even temporarily, to give you some reprieve. Engage in an activity that your brain needs to focus on. Something as simple as a wordsearch, crossword or a jigsaw all need concentration. I often do a weights session because when I lift weights I have to bring my sole attention to that so I don't injure myself.
- **Talking yourself out of the spin** – try telling yourself the reality of the situation – for example, that the person you messaged who hasn't responded yet isn't ignoring you, it's because they're busy, or the phone rang just as they were going to reply, or they haven't had the time to look properly yet. If you insist on that being the actual story, rather than the negative one, it takes back your power and sense of control.

Talking yourself out of the spin

Take a moment to reflect on the dominant thoughts that are swirling in your mind right now.

Write down the five main ones. They can be related to anything: health, career, relationship, family, etc.

Now go through each of the thoughts, and for each one, ask yourself, 'Is this a fact?'

Always look for the evidence. Without evidence, these thoughts can be merely stories you have conjured up in your mind.

Actively challenge your thoughts and then look for alternative explanations to replace the existing thoughts.

Neuroplasticity

The science behind the idea of learning how to change our way of thinking is fascinating, particularly the theory of neuroplasticity.

Has someone ever told you that 'You just need to change the way you think'? That can be an incredibly frustrating and reductive thing to hear, especially if you don't know how. Sometimes it can feel that it's a line someone says simply for the sake of it, rather than providing you with useful advice to achieve something meaningful.

But the good news is that we *can* change our thinking.

This is down to the concept of neuroplasticity, which is the brain's ability to adapt, change, reorganize and grow neural pathways. *Neuro* refers to the neurons, the nerve cells which are the building blocks of the brain and the nervous system. *Plasticity* refers to the brain's ability to change.

Rewiring your brain might sound complicated, but it's

absolutely something you can start to do yourself. When your brain's circuits get caught in negative narratives, your thoughts can skew towards the negative. It is possible to move beyond negativity by paying more attention to the positive aspects of your life.

Reframing negative thoughts

Take five minutes to intentionally recall some of the thoughts you have had in your head today about your fears, your worries, your stressors.

Write these thoughts down in one column.

Now in a separate column counteract each one of the above thoughts with a positive memory.

If you fear failure, write down a time when you have had a valuable lesson from failure. If you are stressed about exams, write down a time when you did well in an exam. It will help to reframe your mindset to move beyond the negative thought loop.

The important thing to remember is how you respond in the 'counteracting column'. You don't want to replace your initial thought with something that isn't truthful or realistic.

If you want to think in a more positive way, you need to consistently reinforce that behaviour. It will take time and consistent practice – doing it once or twice will not result in lasting changes. Your thoughts are fundamental in helping you cope with stress and creating wellness in your life. The way you think impacts your emotional state, which then impacts the chemicals in your brain. Positive thoughts can lead to feeling better – physically and mentally.

Try these simple steps each day to begin cultivating positive thoughts:

- **Affirm positive statements to yourself out loud or in your head** – create your own positive affirmations, write them down where you can easily access them and go back to them every day. Leading performance and health coach Gerry Hussey recommends reciting positive affirmations as part of your morning routine.
- **Keep your goals realistic, but challenging** – they should allow you to push yourself and grow. If the desired result is too easy to attain, you may be less motivated as you could become bored when you know you can achieve it without too much effort.
- **Write down three things that you want to be more aware of throughout each day** – examples include how you speak to yourself, how you speak to others, your body language, your reaction to constructive criticism, how present you are in conversations.

Just a reminder: our brains naturally default to negative thoughts about the future and have a natural negativity bias. Don't be too hard on yourself if your brain jumps to the negative – it's a natural occurrence – just know it's one that, with a little work, you can control and begin to change. That doesn't mean you will always think positively, nor should you place an expectation on yourself to do so, but at least you will be able to get a handle on certain situations and not automatically respond, or think, in a negative way.

Five morning affirmations

- I am enough. I have enough.
- I believe in myself. I can do tough things.
- I do my best, and my best is good enough today.
- I am only getting started.
- I trust myself to make the right decisions.

Accepting our strengths and acknowledging our weaknesses

'Our strength grows out of our weakness'
— Ralph Waldo Emerson

Part of accepting who you are is to acknowledge that you aren't perfect – nobody is. We all have strengths and flaws and these all make us who we are. We need to recognize and embrace our strengths, and these will allow us to work on our weaknesses. It's not easy to accept the negative aspects of ourself, but in accepting them, we also realize that they don't define us.

I think it's so easy to say 'love yourself', but nobody tells you how to do this. It's not something that comes naturally to us. My interpretation of this is simply to be your own ally. I don't mean that you must defend every decision that you've ever made, but rather accept and understand that you might struggle at times.

Accept that you are vulnerable, that you have made mistakes, done things or said things you wish you hadn't. By acknowledging yourself as a flawed person, you open yourself up to change. Click the 'I accept' button on your past. Some say *let it go*, but I say *let it be*. Let the things you can't change stay in the past, learn from those experiences and move forward with more wisdom and knowledge.

The power of identifying your strengths

The sporting arena holds no prisoners. All your weaknesses are on display to the world. While our strengths are acknowledged, it is our weaknesses that are focused on, criticized, analysed. One period during my camogie career particularly sticks in my mind. In 2012, I suffered a bout of bronchitis that took me out of training for a few weeks. When I finally got the all-clear to return, my usual position – wingback, number seven – was now occupied by another player. I was

37

sent up the field to play centre forward, a position much more focused on scoring. The broken windows at the gable end of my childhood house would attest to the fact that I wasn't the most natural scorer.

This move to the forward line threw me. My Cork camogie identity was tied to the number-seven jersey and this change from defence to attack took its toll, both mentally and physically. By playing in a totally different position, the game of camogie as I knew it had changed. In subsequent games I didn't feel like I was able to utilize my strengths and, if anything, the positional change highlighted my weaknesses. It left me feeling frustrated, exposed and totally questioning myself. I went from being an All-Stars award winner in the previous two seasons to getting dropped from the starting team in the 2012 All-Ireland Semi-Final.

I was devastated, but I had to try to separate myself from the negative self-talk. Yes, I had been dropped, but this was the manager's choice and not mine. I had to remind myself that he was making decisions in the best interests of the team and it wasn't my call. So, I made a conscious effort to support my teammates in the run-up to the match and vowed that if I came on as a substitute during the game, I would do my absolute best. I would put the team first. I came on in that Semi-Final, we went on to win it and I regained my place for the All-Ireland Final, but again as centre forward.

We subsequently lost that Final, badly. It was gut-wrenching then, and is still a sore spot for me now, even over a decade later. At the time, I couldn't quite find the lesson in my experience: my ego was bruised and my confidence was shaken. But I do know that I tried my best within the circumstances that were presented to me. That was all I could control. I experienced it, I learned from it and subsequently became a stronger player – and person – because of the pain of losing something that was important to me, but I am still here.

Sometimes, listening to other people can help you recognize your strengths and help you develop self-belief. Back in 2006, my Intercounty coach was Fiona O'Driscoll. She was a former Cork camogie star and one of my sporting heroes growing up. During the year, she asked every player to write down one strength they thought each teammate possessed either on or off the pitch which made them an asset to the panel. After doing this, we promptly forgot about it, but the night before the All-Ireland Final, we were staying overnight in a hotel. When we were back in our rooms after dinner and getting ready for bed, a letter was slid under each door with our name on it. The letter contained a list of all the positive comments our teammates had made about us.

All too often in sport, to focus on improvement, we are focused on pinpointing the negatives. But this completely shifted our mindset to focus on our strengths and what positive attributes and skills we all brought to the squad. It was extremely powerful for a lot of us, because we don't allow ourselves to acknowledge our strengths enough, and when your peers recognize and value your contribution, it definitely increases your confidence.

We went out on to the pitch the next day and ripped through the opposition. We didn't give them a sniff of the ball. I was chosen as Player of the Match, and it was one of the best games I've ever played in the Cork jersey. I put this down to the self-belief and confidence I got from the power of other people's words. I often reread that letter in the months after the Final and I still have it today. It provided me with such a confidence boost, and it sparks such positive feelings every time I've read it since that night. I have since learned to harness the positive power of my own words too, not just the words of others.

We need to realize that it's okay to acknowledge our strengths and recognize how we can bring them to the table in all aspects of life. When I work with corporate groups, I do an exercise where they walk over to a person they don't know and say 'One of my strengths is . . .' It's useful to be able to acknowledge that you are capable, you are talented, and you can use your strengths to develop self-belief and progress to where you want to go in life, even if you find it a little uncomfortable at the start.

What are *your* strengths and weaknesses? Do you know? Think of a time you were really satisfied or a time you were proud of yourself – why were you proud? Be objective and write down the things you are great at and the things you could improve in.

If you can figure out some of the answers to those, and also accept that we are constantly growing as people, constantly discarding memories and making new ones, you can shape a self-image that you feel good about.

What is your USP?

To go a step further, take time to think about your USP. Your USP is your 'unique selling point' and is the essence of what makes you stand out amongst others. It's a marketing term for products and services, but I apply it to people too. It's what differentiates you from the rest. How are you different and unique? What makes you a valuable asset?

When I worked in recruitment years ago, nothing made interviewees squirm more than the question 'Why should you get the job over everyone else?' If you don't know your USP, how can you expect others to know? You could have hidden strengths, skills or attributes that you are too shy to openly show or share, in case people think you are boasting, cocky or have 'notions'.

Maybe you are good at thinking calmly and rationally in a crisis. Perhaps you are able to stand back from a situation, assess it objectively and offer alternative solutions. You might have brilliant persuasion skills or be a talented public speaker.

Invest the time to figure out your USP. It can be your secret weapon, and please don't be afraid to use it.

3. Don't compare, don't despair

'When you are content to be simply yourself, and
don't compare or compete, everyone will respect you'
— Lao Tzu

I don't think it's just me when I say that social media, for
all its positives, has created a world in which we are always
comparing ourselves to each other. It often causes us to frame
our lives in terms of what we don't have, rather than what we
do have. While I think it has always been human nature to
look at what someone else has, or what they are doing, social
media has just made it more immediate and intense. We lie in
our beds before we go to sleep, stand in the kitchen making
dinner, sit in our living rooms half watching TV, always on
the phone, scrolling and scrolling through images and reels
of other people's perfect lives.

And we all do it, we all compare ourselves to others in
every facet of our lives – from how we look to what we're
wearing, our houses, our jobs, our families. We're constantly
measuring our success against someone else's. Exhausting,
right?

Allison Keating, psychologist and author of *The Secret Lives of Adults*, has a useful technique that can help unlock self-confidence, especially when it comes to comparing ourselves to others. Allison revealed that many of her clients, despite being exceptionally accomplished, still lack belief and confidence in themselves – nobody is immune to these feelings of self-doubt. She suggests that we should imagine the 'breadcrumb trail' in order to figure out when our mood began to change to a more negative one.

It can be hard to pinpoint at the beginning, but with some reflection you can start to notice when you first began to feel upset or frustrated in yourself. It may have been after scrolling through social media feeds when you compared your body shape to an image of another person, or when you saw someone, maybe someone you don't even know, achieving something that you would like to do. In that moment the comparison may have led to a break in connection with your authentic self. With no real 'behind the scenes' insight, you put that person on a pedestal, simply because they *appeared* to be 'picture perfect'. For all you know, they too could be feeling the exact same way about someone else.

Remember, confidence is an inside job: it is about exploring, understanding and then accepting your unique self. That's the key to unlocking real confidence. It is cultivated from the relationship you have with yourself.

It is difficult for acceptance and comparison to happily coexist. We cannot fully accept ourselves for who we are if we are constantly measuring ourselves up against other people. Comparison has an annoying habit of tricking you into thinking you're not good enough, not smart enough, not happy enough – not worthy. It makes you lose sight of your talents, your value and your worth. Comparison is inextricably tied up with the idea of failure and negative self-talk. Instead of acknowledging how smart, capable and strong we are, we spend our time comparing our failings against others' successes. This comparison game leaves you feeling like a failure, and can manifest itself as stress, anxiety, sadness and even depression.

A bruised ego, and a lesson learned

A few years ago, I was an ambassador for a cancer charity, and I was asked to take part in a big charity run in Phoenix Park. I signed up for the 5km run (luckily having the presence of mind not to sign up for the 10km run!) and, standing at the starting line, my nerves began to hit. While I was fit and strong, I wasn't a runner. I sprint in camogie, just short, sharp bursts, but I didn't have any training for longer distances.

I was standing there in my leggings and charity T-shirt, ready to go, and as I glanced around at my fellow runners, they looked so professional. They were decked out in their singlets, running shorts, top-of-the-range runners, the fancy watches to track timings and distances. Suddenly I wondered what I had signed up to. I didn't realize at the time, but they were the long-distance endurance athletes, just out to support a charity run. They were used to running marathons, so a 5km run was the equivalent of a warm-up for them.

The photographer asked for a photo of me leading the

pack as the run started, so that's what I gave him – 3,2,1 . . .
I was off at a blistering pace. But then the competitor in me
committed the cardinal sin of running tactics – I kept going
at that pace, determined to keep up with the professionals.
It wasn't long before I realized there was a high possibility
that I was going to get sick or collapse, or both. As I tried to
battle deceptively slow, steep inclines, I became increasingly
demoralized as people passed me by. I wanted to stop, to
look for the nearest ditch and dive into it. I thought about
feigning an injury – maybe a pulled hamstring or a twisted
ankle. But I somehow carried on, the last kilometre feeling
like 24 kilometres, and I passed the finishing line right into
the waiting arms of a camera crew.

I had never fully understood the phrase 'smiling through
gritted teeth' until I had to do that interview, having to
remember key lines about the charity, when I felt like such
a failure inside. I wasn't right for days after that experience,
I was in bits physically and suffering from a severely bruised
ego. Even though I had run faster than I ever had, achiev-
ing a personal best and shaving minutes off my time, I still
gave myself such a hard time. I had spent the entire race
comparing myself to those endurance runners when I'm not
an experienced runner. It was a valuable lesson – I allowed
myself to get distracted by other people when I should have
focused on myself and the reason why I was taking part in
the race.

I know now that I shouldn't have felt like a failure because,
first, I wasn't there to win; second, I was taking part in a
charity event; and third, I did really well. I should have been

enjoying it, meeting people and just having fun while raising awareness for the charity. Instead, I put so much pressure on myself by comparing myself to people who had trained for months or years. My head spun a negative story in which I made a show of myself and everyone passed me by. All I could focus on was how everyone was going to talk about the charity ambassador who couldn't even run.

If you have to compare, be realistic!

If you do insist on comparing yourself or your performance with others, at least compare like with like. For example, if you are learning to cook don't compare your lemon drizzle cake or Sunday roast with someone who has been to culinary school and is super competent in the kitchen.

This is particularly important when you are starting anything new, so that you don't feel deflated and give up before you have hardly begun. You might be in the first chapter of your new story, so don't ruin the experience by comparing it to someone else's chapter 30.

So, how do we stop comparing ourselves in a negative light and learn to embrace ourselves for who we are and what we are able to do or achieve?

46

Curate who you follow

On social media, find someone you admire and follow them. Unfollow the people who you know trigger negative reactions. The first thing I worked on at the beginning of my path to self-acceptance was to stop comparing myself to other women. I found this challenging, because I think it's easy for us to slip into the bad habit of focusing on photos of women we wished we looked like, and especially those images that create impossible expectations and ultimately make us feel bad about ourselves. It's essentially a form of self-sabotage, as we know we will never look like that other person.

When it comes to our abilities, we're all different. The same is true when it comes to our body shapes: we all have different features. Yet we seem to have a much tougher time accepting that fact. Growing up, I was a big *Friends* fan. I used to look at photos of Jennifer Aniston and wished I looked like her. And within the sporting field, many sportswomen in the Irish media at the time, while inspirational in terms of their dedication and success, looked nothing like me in terms of body shape. All I saw were leggy, lean athletes.

I wanted to be like Sonia O'Sullivan when I was younger, but I quickly realized that my body wasn't designed for long-distance running. Then I discovered Serena Williams. Serena's body was her instrument, a machine to propel her to success on the court. She used it to her advantage. The power behind her serve was incredible.

Serena won her first Grand Slam title in 1999 as I was going into secondary school. I was inspired. Like Serena, I played a fast, competitive game, twisting and turning my body, hitting hard, changing direction instantaneously. My body looked like it did because it needed to be strong and muscular to excel in my sport. Just like Serena's.

I also admired how Serena fused fashion and functionality on the court. She experimented with colour and different outfit styles, breaking away from the traditional tennis whites. She was the first sportswoman I had ever seen to wear a jumpsuit on the court and absolutely rock it! She was bold, brave and followed her own path. She owned her body shape and was damn proud of it. She inadvertently instilled in me the courage to try and do the same as I got older. It's still a work in progress.

Embrace the competition

You can use comparison as a motivational tool. Think about the people who inspire you and think about what you can learn from them. It might help you set a target for something you would like to achieve. For example, imagine setting a goal of running a mile loop. You've never run before but you want to get active and healthy.

So, you set out to do it, and your neighbour whizzes by you on her five-mile run. The immediate thought that enters your mind is 'Oh, I'm not as good as she is, I'll never be. What's the point of me even trying?' You go home feeling disheartened. You don't want her to run by you again as you're fearful that she might think you're terrible at running. And so you give up.

Now you've done yourself a disservice. Instead of comparing yourself unfavourably against your neighbour, why not flip it on its head? Why not think 'I can't wait to be able to do that five-mile run too, I just need to build up gradually and try to get out for a run a few times a week.'

Essentially, your neighbour is just doing her own thing, and what she does has nothing to do with you. You can choose to see her effort as a threat or inspiration. Lean in to your feelings of vulnerability and know you won't regret taking this time to improve your life. A day will come when you turn that one-mile slow jog into a five-mile run and a new runner sees you and wonders if they will be able to do that someday.

Identify triggers

We all have certain things or people that cause a negative reaction, and it is important to be able to identify who or what triggers you into a negative spiral of thinking. Does a particular influencer, friend or work colleague make you feel down when you compare yourself to them? A useful thing to do is to write a list of who you compare yourself to. Write down how exactly they negatively impact you, and then think about how this comparison is a waste of your valuable time.

Gratitude journal

The only person you should be comparing yourself to is you. Embrace yourself from within and remind yourself of the positive things about you and your life. Taking a moment each day to sit down and reflect on a few things that you are grateful for can help to focus your mind on the good things in your life. It helps you to step away from unfavourable comparisons. Commit to writing regularly at a certain time of the day and honour the commitment. You might be surprised to see how much it can help!

4. Embrace the body you're in

'Being a healthy woman isn't about getting on a
scale or measuring your waistline. We need to start
focusing on what matters – on how we feel, and how
we feel about ourselves'

– Michelle Obama

A lot of what I think about self-love isn't just about embracing
all aspects of my character and who I am as a person. It's about
loving the body that I inhabit. I think it's safe to say that we
all struggle with accepting aspects of our body. It's hard for us
to love our cellulite, our stretch marks, a rounded tummy, a
wrinkled forehead, when we are constantly bombarded with
images of feminine perfection in the media.

We are constantly fed the lie that make-up, cosmetic
surgery, new clothes and weight loss will make us look good
and will make us feel good. But I think we all know that any
benefit we may get from any of those things is only fleeting.
When you learn to value your body for what it can do, rather
than what it looks like, you are engaging in an act of self-love.

It's not just the media that can cause us to struggle with
body image. Throwaway comments from people around us

can trigger us into a negative spiral. I can remember exactly where I was and what I was doing the first time someone commented on my body – a comment that I perceived negatively and carried around with me for years. I was fourteen years old and hanging out with some friends, as you do, down the town after school, slagging each other and laughing, having a good time. I hadn't thought much about how I looked, I was just wearing a hoody and a pair of jeans and runners, typical teen fashion back then. 'Well, Anna,' one of the lads said, 'I wish I had your legs, they're so strong.'

It was a casual remark, he meant nothing by it. But I looked down at my legs and, for the first time in my life, I saw my body in a different way. We were all sporty, we all knew the benefit of strong legs, and I think he thought I would take it as a compliment. But all it did was make me self-conscious about my body for the very first time.

Despite the casualness, despite the good intentions, despite everything that came after for me – all the good stuff, all the times lads chose better words for their compliments – that *one* sentence stayed in my mind and, I'll be honest, it still does to a certain extent. Even now, despite myself, whenever I scrutinize my body, in the mirror while out clothes shopping, or in photos or on TV, my eyes are instantly drawn to my legs.

I think all women have such stories. Those moments when we realized that we were supposed to look a certain way. The times we realized that maybe we didn't conform to the rigid idea of femininity that society dictates, and that we all fall short of. A throwaway comment can cause a lifetime of negative focus.

When I started to become aware of my own figure, the

trend was to be super skinny; the term 'heroin chic' was everywhere. The fact that women were supposed to model their bodies on something so destructively negative is mind-blowing. And even now, when we hear someone say 'you look thin' or 'you've lost weight', we celebrate – being skinny is almost a social currency that buys approval.

Even appreciating the power that my body gives me, I still often want to change how it looks. I, like so many, am not immune to the pressures placed on women's bodies by society. They are deeply ingrained in us. Looking back now, when I was at my slimmest, I was not necessarily at my healthiest. When society continues to tell us we should look a certain way, it's hard not to at least *wish* we could.

This myth propagated by the media of what we should look like is not only unrealistic but is incredibly damaging, both mentally and physically. It is unattainable. When we see celebrities with the 'perfect' body, we don't know the reality of what went into achieving it – the long hours spent in the gym, the personal trainers, the private chefs and specialist dieticians. Not to mention the best cosmetic surgeons, stylists and make-up teams on speed dial.

The challenge for girls and women – they should be appealing

For me, the most important thing to focus on is body health – not body image. We need to restore the balance towards health. We have to reframe our idea of what a healthy body actually is and it is not necessarily a skinny one, it is one that is fit for purpose and strong.

A few years ago, I presented a documentary on why girls quit sport and I saw how much pressure girls are under. I asked a group of inactive teens why they didn't play sport. One of their reasons was that they didn't feel confident in sports gear. They were conscious of being sweaty and feared being judged about how they looked when running around.

You might roll your eyes but give the girls a break – it's not vanity on their part to think they'll be judged: that is the reality. Women are told from an early age to be ladylike, not to run around, not to fight, not to ruin their clothes. We are literally instructed in the art of appeal. How can we blame each other for falling in line? I have seen first-hand the difference between the reporting on men and women in sport. The commentary about women is often about how they look, rather than what they can do.

I wish the world would reframe things for women. I wish it would stop pushing the ideal of girls as being fragile when we know they are not. We know girls and boys are equally capable of being strong and fierce. I wish the world would stop valuing women on how we look over what we do.

Getting beyond self-consciousness

I can't say 'I did it, so you can too', about ignoring negative remarks, because the truth is that, even though I played sport, I was still hit with the self-consciousness and upset of being judged for my body rather than my prowess on the pitch. Even with the supportive parents, coaches and team that I had, there were so many times when I made bad choices based on impossible beauty standards. I have been guilty of giving the critics far too much power over how I feel; I have handed over my sense of self to other people, even to anonymous trolls on the internet.

Being self-conscious impacted me throughout my career, so I know exactly the damage it can cause. I've dabbled in the fad diets and exercise trends. As a result, I've experienced the negative impact of self-consciousness, both physically and in the emotional relationship I've had with my own body. If I have one regret about my time on *Dancing with the Stars* it's not that I could have danced better, or committed more, but rather I wish I had accepted my body for how brilliant it was.

I look back at pictures now and, honestly, I want to have a strong word with my past self, because on reflection I realize how hard I was on myself. When I looked at myself in the various costumes, I couldn't fully appreciate at the time how stunningly beautiful they were, the intricate details, the colours, the materials. I was focused only on how they looked on me. Were they too tight in a certain place, too short, too revealing? Looking back, I realize now that I wasn't just fit, but aesthetically – based on mainstream ideas about appearance – I was in the best shape of my life. Yet, I wasn't content. I wanted to look even better and I put myself under such pressure. After all, I was the sportsperson, so I needed the audience to see a super-fit, lean body.

I distinctly remember standing in the wardrobe department

with tears in my eyes as I was shown some of my costumes. I wish I could have taken a step back to celebrate my body for what I was putting it through, how it was supporting me through my rigorous dance training, and also acknowledge that I looked great in the outfits as I tried them on. I didn't appreciate how fit and healthy I looked. I guess I felt pressure (mostly from myself) to look better. Whatever 'better' was meant to be.

And now, I often think about the countless girls (and women) sitting in the stands and watching from the sidelines, all across Ireland, who should be taking part in sport themselves, but feel too self-conscious to do so. Maybe some could be Olympians or All-Ireland champions, but all could be participants. I can't help but get angry because this problem is caused by the way we continue to analyse and judge the girls and women who engage in physical activities and sport.

So, what can we do? How can we change our own thinking about our bodies to reframe it for ourselves, and hopefully for our children?

Recently, I found the answer. Acceptance. Self-love. Knowing my own worth – as a woman, as a sportsperson, a friend, a daughter, and now a mother – as something more than just my body.

Our bodies are instruments, not ornaments

Accepting how we look doesn't mean we shouldn't ever want to improve ourselves. It's why I have reservations about the body positivity movement and what it represents. Body positivity is based on the idea of loving who you are, as you are. But it still places the emphasis on how our bodies *look* and opens the way for people to freely comment on others' bodies. I'm not sure if pointing out cellulite, stretch marks, excess body fat, is true body positivity. We are still drawing attention to visual aspects of bodies. Yes, all those things are normal, but why highlight them or comment on them at all?

I think a better way forward is to aim for what is being called 'body neutrality' – in other words, simply accepting your body as it is, trying not to get emotionally caught up with how it looks, one way or the other. We are more than just our bodies. We are complex beings with our own distinct personalities, emotions, hopes and dreams. Body neutrality allows us to appreciate what our bodies do for us every day – take our dogs for walks, play sports, engage in hobbies, do the food shop – rather than focusing on how they look.

While body positivity is well-motivated, and has been a corrective to decades of unrealistic and unhealthy expectations about how we should look, it can leave many of us nervous about admitting that we want to improve ourselves. Improved levels of health and fitness aren't about numbers on the scales and never, ever about size. We can want our bodies to be at their best and move forward in that mindset instead of forcing ourselves to accept (or pretend to accept) what we don't want. Striving for health and fitness and the best for our bodies in a spirit of neutrality is good for both physical and emotional health.

There is so much to unlearn when it comes to our bodies,

because of what we have been exposed to for decades. Not punishing or starving our bodies in the run-up to big events or holidays. Not 'earning' our weekend takeaway. Not referring to ourselves as 'bold' for having dessert. All because we feel we need to be smaller, thinner, slimmer, skinnier, *insert word of choice here*.

We can tell ourselves 'I'll be happy when . . . I am that size' or 'when the scales say X' or 'when I drop the baby weight', the list goes on, but you will not automatically love yourself when that day comes, if it ever does, because you will already have damaged the relationship you have with your body.

Throughout this book you will see that I place a great deal of emphasis on the power of language, and how what we say to ourselves and others can leave a lasting imprint on the relationship we have with ourselves, particularly with our bodies. Words like *syns*, *cheat meals*, even *good* and *bad* foods, reinforce a negative relationship with our bodies – and, quite frankly, with food.

If we see our body as an ornament for other people, we will never find peace with it. But if we see our body as our instrument to live, then we will want to maintain it. It's a different mindset. The goal is an unwavering, unconditional self-acceptance, and we should always keep pushing in that direction. We might not get even halfway there but that isn't a failure: even one step in that direction is a win because a win here equates to a more accepting mindset.

Coming close is better than staying where we were.

Choose your hard

It is hard to work on the relationship with yourself, and to challenge your thinking about how you see yourself. It is an uncomfortable and vulnerable place to be. To come to a point of acceptance that there will be parts of your body which you simply cannot change or get rid of, to understand they are a part of you, and in it for the long haul with you, can be difficult. We all need to get to a place where we realize that we don't need to love every inch of our bodies, just simply accept those parts regardless. You still need to work with your body and not against it. You are in this journey together. You need to be your body's ally, not its enemy. That is a hard destination to reach.

But do you know what else is hard?

Tearing yourself apart, day after day. Wasting energy, wishing that you looked different. Ignoring the impact of genetics, your environment and the many other reasons that contribute to you looking the way you do, and then pressing the 'destroy' button on your body confidence and self-worth.

Many of us have come to believe it's okay to dislike or even hate our bodies. Some may have seen their parents standing in front of mirrors for years picking themselves apart, going on yo-yo diets, or covering up in oversized clothes. That to me is a harder road to travel, because there is no progress to be made on that road.

Both routes are hard. Which hard do you choose?

Consider trying out the following tips to help you embrace your body and practise self-love and acceptance:

- **Engage in physical activity** – it is the most empowering thing you can possibly do. Whether it's an evening stroll, joining a swimming club or going to a weekly yoga class, find the right activity for you and commit to it. It will make you feel good. You will be amazed at what your body can do, and the health benefits are innumerable. Exercise because you appreciate your body, not because you dislike it.
- **Do something that makes your body feel good** – train your brain to associate your body with positive feelings. So go for a massage to ease muscle tension or put your cosy pyjamas on at the end of a hard day, or even just take a long, hot bath. Anything that is pleasurable to your body.

60

- **Don't judge others' bodies** – we always do it, right? Comparing other people's bodies to ours. Evaluating flaws, internally critiquing. But for you to learn to love and accept your own body, you need to stop judging other people's bodies. Bodies are not a valid measure of a person's value. You deserve to be loved and accepted regardless of your body, and so do other people.
- **Avoid the all-or-nothing mentality** – remember I mentioned how easily all-or-nothing thinking gets in the way of self-acceptance in chapter 2 (see page 27)? This is particularly true when it comes to our health and well-being. We sometimes think that being healthy requires unrelenting discipline. We have to be strict about our lifestyle – never eating fast food or sweet treats; never binge-watching TV; never spending hours gossiping with friends; always sleeping for eight hours a night – if we're to belong in the ranks of the healthy. And if we don't buy in fully and do everything right all the time, then we are wasting our time. I am here to tell you that this isn't realistic, practical or fun. Sometimes crashing out on the couch, having a pizza and watching a movie is exactly what you need to meet your well-being needs! Tune in to what you need instead of always doing things you feel you should be doing.

Gratitude exercise

Take a page or get out your notebook or journal.
Stand in front of the mirror and name the parts of
your body and something those parts do for you
that you are grateful for. I have filled in the first one!

I love my . . . *thighs*
Because . . . *they help me to run faster than my
opponent on the field*

I love my . . .
Because . . .

What does 'fit' look like?

As a former athlete, and now a new mother in my mid-thirties, I've started to re-evaluate what fitness means to me. When you think about being 'fit' what comes to mind? Lean? Abs? Athletic? Strong? Flexible?

Being physically fit holds a lot of value in people's lives, mine included, and for that reason alone, the fitness industry is one of the largest in the world. Many people share the belief that if you do enough – there's that word again – exercise, then you get rewarded with the status of being fit, with all the connotations fitness has, like being healthy and looking good.

But how much is enough? Is it the recommended 10,000 steps per day? Is it the World Health Organisation's recommendation of at least 150 minutes of moderate exercise a week? How do we know what works for us?

Steps challenge

Most people have heard that we should take 10,000 steps a day to be healthy. You'll find countless online articles reiterating this. In fact, the 10,000 steps target was created as part of a Japanese ad campaign at the time of the 1964 Tokyo Olympics. Marketers wanted to capitalize on the associated fitness buzz and one clever company promoted the manpo-kei pedometer, which literally means '10,000 steps meter' in Japanese. Since then, this memorable number has been used as the baseline number of steps we should aim to achieve daily.

10,000 steps is a challenging number to hit and often ends up being counter-intuitive – making people feel worse when they can't reach it. So my challenge for you is this: if you want to get fitter and healthier, take note of the number of steps you are currently doing, and try to double it. That will be double the movement you do in a day.

For example, if you are doing 3,500 steps per day now and you hit 7,000 steps, that means you have effectively improved your step count by 100 per cent. You absolutely will reap the benefits.

The abundant benefits of fitness

More often than not, we tend to reduce fitness down to what we look like. While body composition is relevant, it's only one part of fitness. Mental and emotional fitness matter too, and yet are so often overlooked. What about wanting a stronger heart, lower blood pressure, minimizing pain, or improving our balance or mobility? These have nothing to do with how we look, but they matter to how we live. Let's also not forget about the social aspect of fitness – wanting to feel challenged or a sense of accomplishment.

So many pages on TikTok and Instagram show pictures of people who devote their lives to achieving aesthetically driven body goals. Often it can be part of their career to do so, and yet these are the very photos we look at and expect to replicate.

During my time on *Dancing with the Stars*, I felt the pressure of expectation. More so from myself than anyone else. I had a muscular physique, which I had worked hard to achieve over the years as a sportsperson. I remember in week three, for Movie Week, I got the opportunity to dress up as Elsa from

Frozen. It was a real-life Disney Princess moment, and yet in the lead-up to the live show I was consumed by self-doubt, as the skirt part of the costume was see-through. Also, I had to do a handstand during the routine and the dress flipped up over my head at one point, revealing a knicker-like insert underneath.

I was so self-conscious and felt so insecure about my legs being exposed like this on national TV, even if it was only for a few seconds. Some of the other competitors affectionately referred to it as #KnickerGate afterwards when I could laugh about it. Ironically, the night I did the contemporary ballroom dance to 'Let it Go', no one was talking about my legs or the sheer skirt, they were just commenting on the choreography of the dance and the fact that I scored three nines from the judges and topped the leaderboard that week.

It was a false story I had built up in my head, and even though I was in physically great shape, I was also nervous throughout the show about how my body would be perceived. How I could be judged, or commented on, or even ridiculed.

Then, as the weeks went on and I started speaking to people, particularly parents of young girls and younger women, I realized it was important to see a body like mine on the TV. I was fit in a different sense. I wasn't 'skinny'. I was strong, powerful and toned but I also wobbled in parts and did not have the perfect physique we see prized in magazines and on social media.

It got me thinking: at what point can you confidently say you are fit? When you can wear a smaller jean size? Or the scales say you have dropped weight? Maybe it's when you can run 5km in sub twenty minutes? We need to address the pressure, judgement and stress that come with trying to reach these unattainable expectations. Let's redefine what being fit looks and feels like. Let's free ourselves from chasing the stereotypical image of being fit and focus on how we can feel better from moving, fuelling our bodies and changing our mindset.

Here are some suggestions to help you focus on fitness rather than appearance:

- **Think about all the things your body does for you** – now and over the years – and write down at least five of them.
- **Set a realistic goal and hit it** – for example, *I will walk the kids to school every day instead of driving.*
- **Don't compare yourself to others** – if you aimlessly scroll social media and base your own fitness goals on what you see others achieving, you will not be successful in your own goals. You need to identify what is good for you and what's achievable for you according to your own personal circumstances. Don't compare yourself to a former version of yourself either. Just focus on the here-and-now. One step at a time.
- **Know what works for you** – with physical fitness, you can excel in one type and struggle with another, so you need to broaden your perspective when you talk about being fit. People can have different levels of fitness in various categories. If you asked me to

66

sprint, my competitive instincts would kick in. But if you asked me to run 10km, I would find it a lot more difficult. However, that doesn't mean I'm not fit. We all have strengths and weaknesses when it comes to exercise and fitness (just like in life), so that's why finding something that suits you, your abilities, skillset and interests is vital for long-term success and enjoyment!

Really appreciating what your body is for!

There will always be times when we need to take a step back and readjust how we see ourselves. I learned this in the most immediate way possible when working on this book, so this comes from the heart!

During pregnancy, especially at the beginning, I struggled to adjust my mindset when it came to my constantly changing body. Often I stood in front of the mirror and didn't recognize my own body. For almost two decades I had been training it for performance – or at least for one form of performance, to be as fit as possible – and suddenly it was doing things outside of my control.

Of course, I was grateful that my body was capable of doing such wondrous things to help my baby to develop but, to be honest, for the first few months I couldn't fully accept the changes and was quite daunted by them. I realized my goal had to change and, though I was overjoyed to be pregnant, it took a while to really embrace what was happening.

That just shows you how conditioned we are in our view of our bodies and what they are for.

I'm sharing this because I know I'm not the only woman to have felt like this and to fear being criticized for admitting it. Because, let's face it, not only do we have to deal with our bodies being judged, but also our feelings about our bodies being judged – we can't win! The general view is that we should just be grateful to be pregnant and there isn't much room for talking about struggling with the changes. But mixed feelings about our bodies are normal for many if not most women and pregnancy hormones don't magically turn them off. I hope sharing that I found it challenging is helpful to some women.

The same is true – in reverse – post-pregnancy. Now, you are meant to focus on the state of your body, and pronto. We spend forty weeks growing a baby, our bodies undergoing incredible transformations to allow this to happen, and as soon as the baby is born, there is an unspoken pressure about getting our body to 'bounce back' to its pre-pregnancy state. Celebrities' post-pregnancy bodies are widely discussed on social and in other media, with praise for those who appear to 'shrink back' to their 'original' shape quickly and a version of sympathy – which is barely disguised judgement (the implication being: *she mustn't be trying hard enough*) – for those who don't. This type of narrative undermines the marvel of what the body has gone through during pregnancy and birth. Why do we not celebrate the C-section scar in the same vein as we do the return of muscular definition or being able to fit back into a pair of pre-pregnancy jeans?

Now that I'm out the other side of pregnancy – with a lovely baby boy to show for it – I am in awe of the female body and its capabilities. My body was performing spectacularly, just in a different way than I'd ever experienced before!

Valuing your body – a time-travel exercise!

Imagine for a moment if we lived our lives in reverse from a physical standpoint. So, you would experience what it might be like to have a frailer body first, a body that might frustrate you at times, because it couldn't do the things you want it to do – lift heavy shopping bags, put the suitcase into the overhead cabin compartment, get out of a car unassisted.

In those moments would you be thinking about what size your jeans were, how you wished your arms were 'less flabby' or wondering if people were staring at your legs in your shorts?

More likely you would be thinking 'I wish my body could serve me better', 'I wish I could move more freely', 'I wish I was stronger' or 'I wish I could bend down without pain or discomfort'. If you experienced that first, would you look at your body with the same unrealistic standards as you do now?

Our bodies are instruments, not ornaments! Write down all the amazing things that your body does for you. It allows you to walk in the park with your friends, it allows you to bring life into the world, it allows you to climb mountains. The amount of fulfilling, nurturing, practical and enjoyable things it can help you do is infinite.

When you learn to value your body for what it can do, rather than what it looks like, you are on the right path to improving your body image.

The purpose of exercise isn't just about losing inches off your waist. It's about the functional movement of your body. Functional exercises train your muscles to work together and prepare them for daily tasks by mimicking typical movements you might do at home, in work, or during sport or activity.

A squat is a functional exercise because it trains the muscles that you use when standing up and sitting down in a chair, or when picking up an object from the ground. What you do now will impact on your mobility and physical functionality as you get older. Seventy-year-old you will not talk about her thigh gap or six-pack, but she will thank you for investing in her when she can walk up and down the stairs of her house.

Kettle squat challenge

Kettle squats are a tactic I use to incorporate quick bursts of movement into my day. Having a short break in between Zoom meetings? Well, this works a treat.

Think about the following . . .

If I asked you to complete 800 squats in a four-week period, it might sound like an overwhelming challenge that many would shy away from. But when it comes to exercise it's about breaking things down into manageable chunks.

Let's say you boil the kettle three times a day to make a cup of coffee or tea. While the kettle is boiling, commit to doing just 10 squats. This is often 'dead' time as we aimlessly scroll on our phones or daydream while we wait for the water to boil. That quickly adds up to 30 squats in a day. That's 210 squats in a week. After a month, you will have completed over 800 squats!

You could pick any exercise of your choice but it's an easy way to get movement into your day. And the science shows us that not only is movement brilliant for our physical health, it's like 'Miracle-Gro' for our brains too.

5. Tactics board for acceptance

'How you love yourself is how
you teach others to love you'

– Rupi Kaur

Do *you* think you can learn to accept yourself, to love your-self for who you are? I believe you can, because you are a person who deserves to be happy and to live a fulfilling life. We all know we aren't perfect, because life has thrown us into situations that can be challenging and that are difficult to navigate. We can only control our reactions to these situations. We can accept ourselves and learn to tune out the useless external chatter that can sometimes overwhelm us. We can choose to use our strengths and our experiences to move forward positively. We can live our own authentic lives in our own way.

Anna's take-home points

- **Practise self-compassion to live a happier life –** treat yourself with the kindness and respect you deserve. Limit negative self-talk, reframe negative thoughts and be aware of the triggers that can send you into a critical spiral.

- **Accept yourself because you are capable of great things** – acknowledge your strengths and accept your flaws. Use past mistakes or failings as a learning experience.
- **Use comparison to motivate you** – instead of focusing on what you are lacking, focus on doing the important things that bring meaning to your life and allow you to achieve your goals.
- **Love yourself** – by believing in yourself and your capabilities.
- **Accept your body as it is** – focus on health not aesthetics, in order to move towards being the best version of yourself. You are more than 'how you look'.

Read

The Secret Lives of Adults – Allison Keating
Eat, Pray, Love – Elizabeth Gilbert
Awaken Your Power Within – Gerry Hussey
The Top Five Regrets of the Dying – Bronnie Ware
The Happiness Trap – Russ Harris

Listen

Think Like a Monk podcast – Jay Shetty
Happy Place podcast – Fearne Cotton
Unlocking Us podcast – Brené Brown
'Hall of Fame' – The Script

'This is Me' – Keala Settle and *The Greatest Showman* Ensemble
'Go Your Own Way' – Fleetwood Mac

Watch

Good Will Hunting
Babe
School of Rock
Little Miss Sunshine
The Full Monty

Notes

Acceptance – my personal tactics board

....

....

....

....

....

....

....

....

....

....

....

PART TWO

Game Plan for Purpose

6. The pursuit of purpose

'Once you know your why, you have a choice to
live it every day. Living it means consistently taking
actions that are in alignment with it'
— Simon Sinek, *Find Your Why*

I put the Simon Sinek quote at the start of this section – about purpose – because it resonates so strongly with me. The *why* is our purpose, our cause, our *raison d'être*. It is the driving force of our lives. It's the *reason* we get out of bed, the *reason* we do mostly everything we do.

When it comes to purpose, knowing your why helps to inject direction and structure into both your daily life and your long-term plans. It is proven that living your life with a purposeful approach contributes to better physical and mental health. Purpose is about creating meaning in your life – that your life matters and that you make a difference.

However, with purpose also often comes a sense of pressure. There can be an expectation for us to find our life's purpose, or else we may feel we are not living our life to the full. This idea can be overwhelming for many of us. It can stifle us and confuse us even more. Because how do you even know where to start?

Purpose is different for everyone – we all have our own unique set of circumstances that influence us, and different points in our life will cause us to re-evaluate our sense of purpose. For example, two people might have the same career, but one can feel motivated and fulfilled, whereas the other might feel unsatisfied. Tuning in to your own daily purpose allows you to actively live according to your values. It enables you to get up every morning, and to feel you are contributing value to your life and to the lives of those around you. The simplest things can add purpose to your day, and I will explore the benefits of finding your purpose in greater detail in the next chapter.

Finding a sense of purpose, even at the worst of times

During the pandemic (do I even dare refer to this dark time in our lives?!) – like everyone in Ireland, and globally – my world turned upside down. Thankfully, I was still working, but I was living life at a much slower pace. Some days I had very little to do, and I found the lack of purpose to be overwhelming on those days. Because I had nothing to do, I would feel lazy, and then I would feel guilty. It was a vicious cycle of beating myself up because my world had been limited, reduced to the confines of my home.

I quickly realized I wasn't alone in how I was feeling. Increasing numbers of people were contacting me, revealing that they wanted to get fitter but lacked the motivation and purpose to do so. I could relate to that. People who usually walked or cycled to work, went to the gym, trained with a team, were now at a loss as to how to exercise at home. I decided to look at breaking physical activity down into realistic bite-size chunks that would help people to keep healthy in body and mind, and to foster a sense of accomplishment and productivity in their days.

A little boost for the mood proved to be a great distraction during what was such a difficult time for so many. I created the concept of 'Strive for 5' where I would select five exercises and do each exercise for one minute, regardless of fitness levels. I decided to trial some Instagram Live Strive for 5 workouts where people could join me online, for free, and we could work out together. Suddenly it became a regular thing. I scheduled them a few times a week on Instagram, and every week for almost a year I was joined by thousands of people who exercised virtually alongside me, regardless of their age or fitness levels. I also posted the Strive for 5 exercises as reels, meaning they could be done in between Zoom meetings, while waiting for the kettle to boil, or during a scheduled workout time.

In those early days of lockdown, the Instagram Lives gave me a sense of purpose. Why? Because they gave me something to feel passionate about, a sense of direction and a sense of achievement afterwards. I had to prepare, plan and organize each session. I wanted it to be a success, not just for me but for the people who took the time to join in. It gave me a reason, a why. Every week my inbox would flood with messages from participants thanking me for helping them to add purpose into their days. They gained a sense of accomplishment from exercising, so that even if they did nothing else, they felt better for doing something.

The Strive for 5 concept grew from there. What started out as just exercises has now progressed into other areas like Top 5 inexpensive pieces of gym equipment and Top 5 items of workout gear to invest in. My Strive for 5 reels consistently hit over 100,000 views, with some reaching 250,000 views, so it was clearly relatable for people. The Strive for 5 concept made me realize what matters to me, what I need and desire for a full life: a connection to other people, a sense of value in my job and being active.

Over the next few chapters, I will share with you some advice and tips that have helped me over the years, through career changes and big life decisions, to find and shape my sense of purpose. I'm hoping these will help you to:

- Find out who you are
- Map out your purpose
- Set your goals
- Motivate yourself to fulfil your purpose

7. Discovering what you really value

> 'He who has a why to live for can bear almost any how'
> – Friedrich Nietzsche

Your purpose in life is unique to you. We all have our own personalities, experiences, skills and interests that combine to make us who we are, and our purpose is related to all of these. In our busy lives, we often lose sight of what our true purpose is in life. Work, family and social expectations can lead you to feel like you have to compromise yourself in some way. But I am here to tell you that you can still discover your purpose by exploring what brings you joy and dedicating more time to it.

A parable about finding your purpose

First, a little story, inspired by the Greek philosopher Plutarch, which has been told in various forms by the German writer Heinrich Böll, the Brazilian writer Paulo Coelho and in many other versions. It's the parable of the fisherman . . .

Once upon a time there was an investment banker who worked hard and eventually made enough money to retire to a beautiful coastal village. He spent the mornings with his wife and then sat relaxing most days down by a pier where he watched a fisherman take his boat out just after lunch every day and then return in the early evening.

The boat would have three baskets on board, and at the end of the day's fishing they would be full to the brim with fat silver fish that the fisherman would sell easily to waiting restaurant owners and housewives who raced down to meet him as he came back to shore.

One day the banker wandered over as the fisherman was tying up his boat and he asked how long it took him to catch such good fish.

The fisherman replied, 'Only a couple of hours.'

The banker said, 'You should stay out all day, you'd fill those baskets five times over.'

The fisherman shook his head. 'This is enough,' he said.

The banker said, 'But what do you do with the rest of the day?'

And the fisherman smiled and told him that he spent the morning with his wife drinking coffee in the sun or resting in his hammock, the afternoon fishing a little, and the evening having a beer and a game of cards with friends in the tavern.

'I'm an investment banker,' the banker said, 'I can help you. My advice to you is spend a full day fishing and take the fish to market, use the proceeds to buy a bigger boat, and with the proceeds from that you could buy a fleet. Sell directly to the processor and open your own fish supplier business. You'd make a lot of money.'

Then he added, 'You'd have to move to the city, of course.'

The fisherman asked how long all that would take.

'Twenty years,' the banker said confidently.

'But what would I do then?' the fisherman asked.

'Well, once your business was big enough you could announce an IPO and sell stock to the public – you would make millions.'

'Millions?' The fisherman stroked his chin. 'What would I do with millions?'

'Retire!' said the banker. 'You could sell up, move to a coastal village, spend the mornings talking to your wife or resting in your hammock, in the afternoon you could fish a little, and in the evenings you could have a beer and a game of cards with friends in the tavern.'

Finding your why is deciding on the life you want to lead and just going for it. Does that make sense? Take the fisherman: he knew what he wanted and wasn't willing to work himself to the bone on the promise of some fantasy future retirement, when he could just carry on enjoying what he was already doing. The businessman was convinced that his drive and ambition in life was for money and a successful business, but the truth was that his goal was the same as the fisherman's. In expending all his energy trying to be a success measured by wealth, he delayed living the life he possibly could have had years before.

The reason I am telling you this story is because I want you to be clear about the life you want, the person you want to be – now. Strip away the stress, the mundanity and the busyness of day-to-day life, and think about what you need to do today to get you closer to living the life you want. Focus on what you have, what you have already achieved in life so far, and it will shape where you want or need to go. It will lessen your fear that you haven't exploited the full potential of your life so far, because you will be able to acknowledge how far you've already come. Think back to a time when what you wanted was possibly what you have right now.

Life purpose statement

Take some time out of your day to sit down and write out a mission statement of the purpose of your life.

What inspires you?
What motivates you?
What are you naturally good at?
What are your values?
Visualize what's most important to you.

Busy, busy, busy

Have you ever found yourself replying to the question 'How are you?' with any of the following: 'I'm up the walls/I'm snowed under/I'm flat out/I'm up to my eyes'? Why is that? Being busy isn't an accurate response to that question, but it's often our default. We assume that if people think we are busy, they may think we are successful, important, indispensable. We wear 'being busy' as a status symbol of sorts. We need others to see, or at least assume, that we are productive with our time, and very much in demand.

Amidst the busyness, we might not get to pause for breath, to take the time to connect with what happiness is for us. If we keep feeding ourselves the narrative that we are busy, we may just start to believe it. This notion of being busy also serves to deny us the chance to reflect on what our true purpose is. Being busy is not a purpose, it's a state of being, and it causes us to forget what would make us happy and fulfilled in life.

Constantly telling people you are busy may result in you missing out on new opportunities. People won't ask or include you because they'll think 'they are too busy'. You might miss out on something that you would have loved to do.

The courage to figure out what you really want

We knew what happiness was when we were children, we knew what our passions were, even if they were ever-changing. We had collections of fancy paper, of marbles, of teddies and favourite toys. We could give answers to most life questions at the drop of a hat. We knew we had to go to school to learn, we knew we had to show up for training once we joined the team, but we also knew our favourite colour, our favourite sweets, and we were fully focused on who we were.

Where along the way did we lose that ability to find happiness in simple pleasures? Is it that we focus on 'success' too much as we shift into adulthood and start aiming for things that might not even matter to us, simply because they are deemed to be signs of success? Do we hear other people talking about buying a house, getting a promotion, and feel we *should* want those things? What if you don't? Are you courageous enough to go against the grain and look for something different, because it is what *you* want?

Should versus Want

Anytime someone tells you what you *should* be doing, replace the word *should* with *want*. They might be telling you what you *should* do – settle down, get married, have children – but ask yourself if this is what you *want* to do?

By doing this, it makes decisions easier.

When I left my business career working for multinational companies after seven years, I decided to go freelance to explore the world of media. People had so many opinions about what I *should* be doing. Most of them had good intentions when giving their unsolicited advice. I'll never forget standing in the kitchen of my friend's house when her dad came in and started talking to me about my recent 'career move'.

'So, you left your pensionable job?' he remarked. 'You could have stayed in that company for the next thirty years.'

That prospect didn't exactly appeal to me. The security that he saw in a pensionable job was a priority in his mind, but it wasn't what I saw.

I explained to him what I was doing instead in my career and, while interested, he still looked confused. Then he said, 'Okay, but when are you going to go back and get a *solid* job?' I simply laughed in reply. He had this idea in his head of what I should be doing, but I knew that it wasn't what I wanted. When I left my business career, I knew that, while it was a good job, it wasn't a good job *for me*.

The simple pleasures

Having passions and having purpose gives us a strong structure for making choices. We find a driving force, or in some cases a reason for 'pressing pause'. The simple joys we found in leaning in to who we were as children still exist in adulthood, we just need to take the time to look.

What we learn from the parable of the fisherman and the businessman is this: we don't need more than what fills our lives with contentment, and we should seek happiness now. How many times have we promised ourselves that we will make that leap, only to revert to what we have always been doing, living on autopilot mode, never making any lasting changes? We all want to feel like we are 'winning at life' so why then are we not even willing to get involved in the game?

You see, each of us is entitled to live a full life. A life that we get satisfaction from, one that we want to live, one that excites us. For some people, life has that tingling excitement that most of us only feel on our way to the airport for a holiday. But why can we not feel like that about our working life, our family life, the day-to-day? What would you say if I told you that it is possible in some capacity?

Feeling fulfilled isn't something for someone else, it's for you. You deserve to live that life. You just need to figure out what exactly it is that makes you feel that way and mould your life around that.

Oprah's Five-Star Pleasures

We need to take the time to shine a spotlight on our lives. To see what illuminates us and how we can hold on to it. Oprah Winfrey often speaks about what she calls Five-Star Pleasures. Small moments that create pockets of happiness in her daily life and fuel her sense of purpose.

For Oprah, it's sitting under an oak tree reading the Sunday papers or being able to do good things for people. For me, it's having a good natter on the phone with a friend, setting the world to rights. It's watching a film with Kev, munching popcorn and Maltesers. It's finding the sweetness in the mundane, it's sharing thoughts and lives – these are my magic moments.

Can you identify what your Five-Star Pleasures are? Take a minute to write down a list. See if you can incorporate at least one into your daily routine.

Who am I?

Asking the question 'Who am I?' takes guts. It's one of the most complex questions you can seek the answer to, but once you figure it out, it forms the basis for finding out what gives you fulfilment and purpose in life going forward. We are the products of our upbringing, the sum of our experiences, and we all have a unique set of values. We are constantly evolving as people, but when chasing a sense of purpose, we need to try to develop an awareness of who we are and who we want to be, and then try to close the gap between these two people.

Identify your values

Our personal values are like an internal compass and will help us discover who we are and explore what might give us purpose. They help determine our priorities and can be the measuring tool we use to see if life is turning out how we want it to. Each of us has our own set of values. You may not be consciously aware of your values, but they do exist. You need to drill down and be as specific as possible when trying to identify yours. Have you ever done something, heard something or said something that just didn't sit right with you? That may be because it conflicted with your values.

Our value systems are first established when we are very young. They can be influenced by our home environment, religious, ethical and cultural beliefs, and life experiences. Maybe you had a sick parent growing up, so health became a shared value in your home, and as you've gotten older you have maintained the importance of taking care of your health. We are often predisposed to adopt the values of our family, so you need to make sure that you hold these values in the same regard as those who instilled them within you.

Our values are the things that are most important to us. Our core values go a step further and are our priority values. These values are at the core of who we are, and when we are in tune with them, they can determine how we handle specific situations. Often, we muddle through life without ever considering our authentic selves, who we truly are, but we are *not* just what we do.

It's quite daunting to explore who we are.

Many of us might worry that we may not like what we find. We do things according to what feels right or easy at the time, and sometimes, in living that way, we lose out on staying true to our values, which can make us feel out of sync in our lives.

For example, if honesty is something you think you value, fact-check this. Are you honest with yourself? Think about it. Are you honest with others no matter what the repercussions may be? If the answer is 'sometimes', or 'no', then your so-called values and who you are do not align. When you hear someone say in the films 'What do you stand for?', this is what they mean. We *think* we know what our values are. But how can we, if we never invest the time in really understanding them?

So how do you find out what your values are?

> ## Questions to ask yourself to discover your core values
>
> - Think of the most meaningful moments in your life. What made them meaningful?
> - What people inspire you? Describe their traits – what makes them inspiring?
> - Identify the times when you were happiest. Find examples from both your career and personal life.
> - Identify the times when you were most proud. Why were you proud?

> - Identify the times when you were most satisfied. Why did you feel satisfied?
> - Think of times when you completed something but still didn't feel satisfied. Why was that?

Using your values to map a route forward

Through doing this exercise myself – figuring out my core values – I have discovered that two of them are *connection* and *legacy*. A famous quote (often attributed to poet and activist Maya Angelou) comes to mind: 'People will forget what you said, people will forget what you did, but people will never forget how you made them feel.'

This is a mantra I come back to again and again. From a legacy perspective I want to leave my stamp on the world, I want to achieve things that will be remembered, but while doing so I want people to remember me for how I made them feel.

It is important to me that people feel good after interacting with me either in the course of my work, my broadcasting, my coaching, or even after a random encounter in the local shop. I want people to feel energized and motivated in my company. I want them to feel encouraged. I want my actions and words to be positively impactful on others I engage with, and I continually work on that, while striving to leave my mark on the world in some way.

96

For the first part of my life, in my teens and twenties, being the best I could possibly be as a camogie player formed a key part of my purpose. When the team was being named before a match, I would be a bundle of nerves and would almost convince myself that I wasn't going to make it. I think a big reason for the nerves was that if I was dropped from the team, I knew I would lose my sense of purpose.

Camogie was such a huge part of my life for years, I felt like it formed part of my identity – it was who I was. Everything else came second. Though I always worked hard at school and obtained a business degree from the University of Limerick, I never felt as if my studies were part of my core *why*. In 2015, when I turned twenty-seven, I cracked my shin bone and couldn't play in the National League. During the time off from playing, I found myself contemplating what my future would look like, without camogie. Camogie made me happy; I loved being part of the team, the thrill of the game, the sense of joy I got on the pitch. But it wasn't sustainable. How was I going to be fulfilled without my beloved camogie? Who would I be without it?

Those thoughts prompted me to begin working on myself – practising self-acceptance, identifying my purpose and my values – and I've never stopped. I identified areas that interested me, and I looked at how I wanted my future self to be.

I have always had an interest in how the mind works, and how people behave, so I looked to my values – connecting to people, wanting to give back – and qualified as an executive and performance coach. Through this I can help people grow and develop in different ways and of course it was invaluable when

I became a coach on *Ireland's Fittest Family*. I had to figure out my own path and using my values as a guide helped me so much in deciding where to go and what to do next. Hanging up on my bedroom wall at the time was a poster with a quote from Ralph Waldo Emerson: 'Do not go where the path may lead, go instead where there is no path and leave a trail.'

I check in with myself now and again to make sure I am living my values and that my values still feel aligned to who I now am and what my purpose is. We are constantly evolving based on life experiences and sometimes our perspectives in life may change, and so our values may need to shift too. But if we don't know what they are to begin with, it can lead to feeling discombobulated – out of kilter with the world and our place in it.

Finding your purpose

Try it on. Does it fit?

We are all striving to find our place, our purpose. You don't have to get it right on the first go. Imagine finding your purpose was like going shopping for a new outfit for an important occasion. You might have to try on a few different ones before finding what works best for you, before you get the feeling that, *yes, this fits – it fits my shape, my personality, my budget, my style.*

The same is true for your purpose. Try it on. Test it out. Question how it feels. In the pursuit of finding your purpose, you may first have to figure out what doesn't fit.

8. Map a route towards your goals

'A goal without a plan is just a wish'
— Antoine de Saint-Exupéry

Having a clear purpose can be transformative. It can enable you to live your happiest, most fulfilled life. How do we fulfil our purpose? By setting goals. Goals are specific, fixed targets that help you achieve your ultimate purpose. Setting goals is a hugely positive thing to do for yourself. It encourages you to make changes and it gives you something to look forward to and to strive towards.

Just imagine . . .

You need to get to a certain location, but you're not quite sure where it is. You've never been there before and you don't know the best route. You would tap open your Google Maps app on your phone, right? You would input your current location and then you'd input your destination point, an address or Eircode, to the exact place you want to be. The app will then plot out the journey, and offer you some options, take you on the scenic route over the side of a mountain maybe (tell me this doesn't just happen to me?!).

Once you've chosen your route and you can see the steps of that journey, it will tell you exactly where and when you need to turn, where you can rest, where you can refuel. Sometimes you may not know what awaits you at the end destination, but you have a clear route for how to get there.

How many of us plot out our lives in the same way?

We can feel more in control when we have a rough route to follow and, even if there are diversions and detours along the way, we still have the directions to get us there in the end.

Goal-setting to achieve our purpose

'The secret of getting ahead is getting started'
– Mark Twain

Setting out clear and defined goals is important because it provides you with a sense of direction and purpose in life. When you set goals, you are consciously identifying what you want to achieve from life, and what you need to do to achieve it. It motivates you to take definite action, and it makes you feel in control of your future. Goal-setting has so many benefits, including how it . . .

- Provides us with a sense of direction and purpose
- Helps to identify what is meaningful to us in life

- Allows us to periodically reflect, re-evaluate and adapt if necessary
- Helps us to stay focused and motivated, especially during setbacks
- Creates accountability
- Fosters a sense of achievement when progress is evident

Goal-setting encourages you to reflect on your life, to make changes where necessary, and it gives you something to focus on and strive for. You need to make sure that what you strive for is attainable in some way, otherwise you will get discouraged, lose focus and abandon the goal.

Be SMART

I have found that when it comes to goal-setting, applying SMART principles is a helpful tool. SMART stands for Specific, Measurable, Achievable, Realistic and Timely. So setting SMART goals helps you to be proactive in reaching your targets. If you put this into practice you will be closer to creating goals that align with your values and who you want to become in life.

Specific   To know we are going in the right direction we need to deal in specifics. We need to know exactly what it is we are aiming to do, and how to do it. If we were building a house we would start with blueprints, right? It's not enough to say, 'I want to build a house,' and to then wander aimlessly around laying bricks and banging nails. We need the exact plans to know the steps to follow. We take those plans and work to build each part from the foundation all the way to the roof, with a clear understanding of what the aim is, what the system is and what the outcome needs to look like. It's the same for our goals in life. If we want to be fit, we need a plan. If we want a new career, we need a plan. If we want to be healthier, we need a plan. Get specific.

Measurable: It's impossible to know if you're moving forward if you don't have a way to track your progress. At the same time, being obsessed with numbers isn't good for anyone. So, deciding how you will track your progress and how often can be a tough thing to decide. However, once you do decide, stick with it. What gets measured gets managed. Checking in and objectively observing (without pressure or emotional attachment) how the plan is working is important in case tweaks need to be made. Otherwise, you could be following a plan that doesn't yield results. Ask yourself what's working and, equally, what's not working. What can happen is that when something isn't working, we tend to give up. But remember, if the plan isn't working, alter the plan, not the goal!

Achievable: Set a goal that is challenging, but still manageable. You want to give yourself every opportunity to succeed, rather than setting yourself up for potential failure. Working towards something that is achievable will boost your confidence and motivation as you will see progress. Progress is the antidote to feeling demotivated. Science tells us that progress pleases the brain, so you can expect a dopamine release when you hit your goal milestones. Dopamine is often called the 'happy hormone'. The flip side is, if your goals are unrealistic, it can cause you to procrastinate and can make you feel overwhelmed.

Realistic: Make sure that your goal is realistic for you. It's not about comparing yourself to anyone else, just focus on yourself. We often think about the end goal, but we need to be aware of where we are coming from too. Think about Google Maps. It's not enough to have an end destination, you also need to know your starting point. Be honest with yourself, it will help to create a realistic goal. Be led by your ambition but be grounded by your reality.

Timely: Your goal needs to have a timeline. By when are you planning to achieve your goal? Then set yourself deadlines to keep yourself on track. The best way to stick to a timeline is to build in some accountability. Studies show we are far more likely to follow through on something if we tell a friend, so get yourself an 'accountability buddy'. Someone that will check in with you regularly, maybe even train with you too, if fitness is a goal.

By making your goals SMART, you increase your chances of success. When things are clear and focused, they become achievable, and when we know when something is due by, we can know how much work to put in and when. Following this goals system can be a game-changer.

The first thing I would suggest is to sit down and follow this SMART plan to work out the goals that align with your values and help you realize your purpose. It is much easier to achieve goals if they are rewarding, rather than money-orientated or to please other people.

For example, if your purpose in life is focused on family, you want to ensure you are fit and healthy to fully embrace this purpose. Your goal is to improve your health and fitness by losing two stone, taking up running and embarking on a healthy-eating plan. Working towards this goal will help you achieve a sense of accomplishment, pride and happiness, especially if it is centred around an activity e.g. if you set a goal to run 2km, you will gain a sense of achievement once you complete it.

Then just start. For some, this is the hardest step. Regardless of where you are at, you can't go anywhere unless you start. You won't know if you can get to wherever you are going until you start. Start small and plan a route, in stages. Note down milestones and aim to reach these one at a time.

The wheel of life

The wheel of life is a coaching tool that I have found useful to help me get a better understanding of my current levels of satisfaction in specific areas of my life. You can use the wheel of life to help you set goals, as it can make it easier to identify the areas that you want to focus on. I like to think that it gives you a helicopter view of your life, as the visual representation helps you to assess the areas to which you want to devote more time, attention and energy.

The easiest way to do it is to take a blank page and draw a circle or 'wheel'. The wheel can be divided up into eight to ten segments that are important in your life, like relationships, health, finance, career, personal development, social life, etc.

Wheel of life

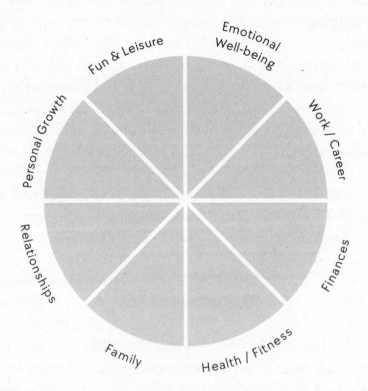

You then rate each aspect of your life between one and ten (one being the lowest) by answering the question: 'How satisfied am I in each of these areas *today*?' Your answer must be based on the present moment. By doing this, you will have a graphic view of where you are now, which will allow you to set goals to get to where you want to be, looking to achieve balance and fulfilment along the way.

Now you need to decide one area you want to start with – you shouldn't try to make changes in all the different areas of your life simultaneously. To make an improvement in your chosen area, ask yourself: 'What small thing can I start doing today to improve the current number by 1?'

Balance in the pursuit of achieving our goals

Many of us want to achieve goals, and still maintain balance in our lives. However, even when we drill down, we are not quite sure what balance looks like, or even what it means for us. We tend to believe that to achieve balance we need to implement huge changes, but the wheel of life can offer you a realistic way to move towards what you want, one step at a time. Nothing drastic but moving at a steady pace.

One thing to keep in mind is something that psychologist Dr Colman Noctor talks about in his book *The 4–7 Zone*. Many of us, regardless of what aspect of life we are shining a spotlight on, either see ourselves in the 1–3 or 8–10 zones. We tend to focus on the extremes, beating ourselves up if we're not doing as well as we 'should' or putting ourselves under pressure to maintain high standards. Or maybe we under- or overestimate how well we are doing or should be doing. Either way, Dr Noctor believes the 4–7 range is the sweet spot to achieving balance and harmony.

With that helpful caution in mind, don't be too hard on yourself if you're scoring low in one of the segments in your wheel of life. A small improvement will make a big difference. And if you think you're doing very well, that's great. But don't get fixated on staying at the top of the range.

Once you are as honest with yourself as you can be about where you are in the various segments on the wheel you can make a plan from there.

The importance of milestones

'Great things are done by a series of small things
brought together'
– Vincent van Gogh

When I was captain of the Senior Cork camogie team in 2014, we came up with collective milestones and we set out to reach those, ignoring the big goals and simply making our way in the direction of our goal by meeting these smaller checkpoints. Instead of making our sole goal winning the All-Ireland Final, we would first aim to get into the League Final. Then win that. Then win the first round of Championship and so on. If we failed to reach a milestone, that gave us a chance to re-evaluate.

Failure can be a great source of feedback if you can detach from the negative emotions that can come with it. It's a chance to reflect and reset. Having lots of small milestones kept us chipping away at the bigger end goal. If we'd had to think about winning an All-Ireland title in September when we were cold and wet in January, running around a mucky pitch, we wouldn't have felt too motivated. However, thinking about the upcoming League milestone in the spring was an easier thing to focus on. If your goal is too far in the distance, in terms of time and achievability, it may become overwhelming and you are less likely to get there. Little milestones do help you to keep focused.

There is something else about this idea that really works: your sense of accomplishment acts like a positive 'success bank'. By the time we got to the All-Ireland Final we had banked a great deal of confidence and self-belief from our cumulative wins that season. We were able to look back at everything that year, all the small milestones we had set out and achieved, and draw strength from those achievements. We were inadvertently carving out a winning mentality.

I strongly believe that if we had aimed only for that elusive All-Ireland title, uncertainty and doubt might have affected our performance. Instead, we had a proven track record from that season to fall back on. There was solid evidence in our success bank that we could achieve such a huge goal.

Marking the milestones

Think of it this way: when you hit a milestone, it works something like a video game (or 'gaming', as it's now called). If you lose a life, you don't go right back to the start, you go back to the previous checkpoint. It works because when you hit the milestone, you know you are capable of success, and when you are challenged along the way and you are struggling to reach the next milestone, those small successes act like reminders, a bank of encouragement to draw from. You know you can do it because you already have. With this approach you have a proven track record. Stick to evidence and facts – you did it before, so go again. Milestones give you a sense of achievement, a boost, that will drive you forward. When you see that you can, you will get there.

It's important to accept that setbacks happen, failures happen, and we will take longer to reach some milestones than others. If we stopped trying something just because we failed the first time or the fifth time, then nobody would ever learn to ride a bike, drive a car, speak a new language. Nobody sits down at a piano and plays Beethoven perfectly – hitting the wrong note teaches you where to place your fingers the next time.

In every match since I was five years old, I have missed the ball or lost it to the opposition on numerous occasions. As players, we need to acknowledge these misses, to address things within the team that aren't working. As a captain, I learned that what gets measured gets managed, even though it can be hard to face up to these things at the time. If you're not reaching your milestone, tweak things, create a smaller milestone to reach, seek support and guidance.

Tragedy isn't the mistakes we make; tragedy is not understanding that if we're to learn we must make mistakes. We have to struggle across that bridge to get to the wonders on the other side.

When setting my goals in life, I have drawn a lot of inspiration from Stephen R. Covey's brilliant book *The 7 Habits of Highly Effective People*. He believes that to bring about genuine and permanent change, we need to undergo a paradigm shift. Well, what does this mean? It means that we need to change our fundamental beliefs and values at a core level, rather than merely adjusting our attitude at a purely superficial level. And in terms of goal-making, we have to 'begin with the end in mind' (Covey's Habit 2). Use your purpose in life to define your goals and use them as a guide to make decisions and prioritize actions.

What is your starting point?

I would say to you, be totally honest with yourself about your starting point. Knowing where you want to go is great, but to plan the route you need to be clear about where you are starting out from. It is key to the successful outcome of your goals. Take the example that I mentioned above, where your goal is to improve your health and fitness. How can you see that happening and how can you move towards that in small ways? What are the baby steps? Yes, it is tempting to go on a strict diet in that situation, especially when you see images and reels on social media promising a quick fix, promising that you can shift a few pounds in days with just a few shakes, but you know from past experience (if not yours, others') that that's not a sustainable change, it's one that will cause more trouble down the road.

Instead, think small steps. For example, switch your daily latte for an Americano with milk. You want to run 5km? Can you currently run 1km? Setting a 5km goal may be unrealistic if you can't yet run 1km. Be realistic with your start point. Ask someone you trust for objective advice on where they think your start point is. Sometimes our emotions can prohibit us from being honest about ourselves.

If there's one thing we can be certain of, it's that we can't predict the future, there are always surprises. But having a sense of purpose and setting goals gives us focus and can even help us realize what we really want. It doesn't mean that we can't change our mind or take a different path or even fall into something else along the way. However, it does give us focus and ideas of timelines, or may even help us realize we want something or we don't. We can't change our past, no matter how many times we reflect on it, but we *can* change our future. Nobody knows what the future holds, but setting achievable milestones is a practice that can change your mind-set and give you purpose.

So go ahead, create your own map in your mind, pin where you are now and pin where you want to be, and make your first move.

Your future self

'Your future depends on what you do today'
– Mahatma Gandhi

We are constantly being told to live in the here and now, be present. But consider this for a moment. We map out and design goals that, we hope, will move us towards where we want to go in life. These goals will help us to change or improve our health, relationships, career. But why don't we spend adequate time thinking and imagining the person we will be in the future, thinking about the life we want to lead?

Some of you may be answering that question with something like 'Well, it's because we can't predict the future. No one knows what it will look like, so it would be hypothetical', and to an extent this is true. However, what is also true is that the decisions we make now impact our future selves and our future lives – whether we choose to believe it or not.

We regularly read articles along the lines of 'what I would say to my younger self', in essence our past selves. But we cannot change our past selves, so let's flip it. If you could talk to your future self right now, what do you think they would say? Would they be pleased with the decisions you are currently making for your future health, well-being, relationships, career? We need to connect more with our future selves so that we can invest in them.

It can be scary to think about the future, especially when there are no certainties. We think about the past because it has already happened and often it's easier to remember than it is to imagine. Your imagination is like a muscle, it needs to be used to be strengthened and developed. Children have great imaginations because they are in regular use. Have you ever bought a toy for a child and an hour later you find them playing with the box that the toy came in, turning it from a racing car to a spaceship in seconds?

As adults, we are conditioned to deal in facts and logic, and using our imagination is often considered daydreaming or simply a waste of time. The assumption is that if it's hard to imagine then it's unlikely to happen. But you need to think about your future self consistently, so that your present self has a map and directions when it comes to making decisions that can help shape your future.

Most of us have thought about our futures at some point. Dr Benjamin Hardy, author of *Be Your Future Self Now*, believes that many people have already assigned themselves default futures. He is of the opinion that many of us don't see our futures being much different to our current lives. Why is that?

Even if we are not happy with where we are now, because it is familiar to us we are willing to stay there rather than seek out something else, as it is unknown. It sounds crazy but it is often the case. What we need to realize is that even if we are not actively trying to change, we still are. The one certainty in life is that we will all change. As the Greek philosopher Heraclitus said, 'The only constant in life is change.'

Visualize to conceptualize to actualize

I believe we need to visualize to conceptualize to actualize. What does this mean? You have to think about what you want your life to look like in the future (visualize), to flesh out the details to develop an idea for your future self (conceptualize), in order to move towards making it a reality (actualize). This will allow you to make decisions and say yes (or no) to opportunities that will take you closer to your future life. You need to be intentional with how you visualize your future self.

Back in 2014, Harvard professor Dan Gilbert did a TED Talk about the psychology of our future self. He spoke about

the decisions we make which can have a profound influ-
ence on our future selves. We live in a world now where
delayed gratification is becoming a thing of the past. No one
is thinking about what our future selves want. Everything is
instantaneous.

Picture these common scenarios. You are watching a new
series on Netflix, one episode ends and you want to know
what happens next, so you just play another episode, perhaps
at the expense of going to bed at a reasonable hour. You've
had a tough day at work, fancy a takeaway? Why wait until
the weekend? Get on to the app and order, and it's here in less
than an hour. If you are in the mood for some retail therapy
but the shops aren't open, fine, just look online. And on and
on it goes. We don't have to wait any more so therefore we
don't want to. The thing is, we can fall into the trap of priori-
tizing what we want to feel now, instead of how we want to
feel in the future.

It is said that an average person makes an eye-watering
35,000 decisions each day.* Daily decision-making as our
present selves can have an impact on our future selves, caus-
ing a ripple effect. As the saying goes, every action has a
reaction.

Another episode on Netflix may mean less sleep. Another
takeaway may hinder your health. Another online purchase
may hamper your saving for that mortgage. All these tiny
ripples taking effect. Now, I am not saying that the above

* Sahakian, B. J., and LaBuzetta, J. N. (2013), *Bad Moves: How decision making
goes wrong, and the ethics of smart drugs*, Oxford University Press.

actions should never be enjoyed (I am partial to all of the above, on occasion even simultaneously) but we do need to make sure that these actions don't negatively impact on who we want to become.

With so many decisions to make every day, many of us can also experience decision fatigue. This can impair our judgement and cause us to make decisions in haste or avoid decision-making altogether. And not deciding is still making a decision. We just remove our involvement and our control. For example, have you ever been asked 'What do you want for dinner?' You can't decide, so you agree to a suggestion in haste or else just say, 'I don't mind,' then when you get your dinner you feel annoyed because you didn't like what was served.

One of the best ways to reduce decision fatigue so that you save adequate energy for important daily decisions is automating processes in your life and creating habits (more on that later). This is why some top CEOs, like Mark Zuckerberg, choose to wear the same clothes to work all the time, or athletes eat the same food every day.

Ask yourself: 'What processes can I add into my daily life to eliminate unnecessary decision-making?'

Create a vision board

A vision board is a visual representation of how you want your life to look. Making a vision board allows you to have a clearer overview of all the different things you want to work towards. Neuroscientist Dr Tara Swart refers to them as *action* boards, a term which I love. When you have a visual representation of your future goals, it may be easier to make decisions that will result in positive actions towards both them and your future self. Here's how to go about it:

- Take some time to reflect on your future goals.
- You can make as many separate vision boards as you want, each with a different focus or theme, or keep it generic about your overall future life.
- You can make a physical board, using a cork board, or a digital version using the likes of Pinterest.
- Look for pictures that represent what you want your future life to look like – career, health, house, nature, car, holidays, partner, children, the list is endless. The more detailed and specific the images can be, the better. Also, be grounded by your reality when making a vision board. The more realistic it is, the more able you are to work towards the outcome.
- It is also important to visualize the process, not just the end goal. For example, if you have a goal to lose weight, and you put up a picture of a dress you want to wear, then also include pictures of the process – fitness, sleep, nutrition.
- Cut out your images and pin them to your board or attach them digitally. Aspirational and motivational quotes and mantras can also be pinned up. You can continually add to the board and remove things as your goals and priorities change.

It is important to put the board where you will regularly see it. Why is this useful? Well, many of us resist change because it is new. When you try something new, the body has a stress response, releasing stress hormones. However, when you repeatedly look at images relating to your future goals, your brain no longer sees them as new, and they seem much more attainable. They become a plan of action, rather than wishful thinking.

9. The engine of change and lasting success – motivation

'I never dreamed about success. I worked for it'
— Estée Lauder

You have identified your purpose, recognized your values, set your goals and established your milestones. But what do you do if it gets a bit tough, if you've had a hard day and you're feeling dispirited? You need motivation! Motivation is your internal drive to achieve your goals, and it's so important to nurture your motivational drive to stay on track and get where you want or need to be.

Motivation is important because it:

- Helps you establish goals to work towards
- Enables you to solve problems
- Helps you to change old habits
- Helps you to cope with challenges

We all have different reasons for needing motivation. It is easier to motivate ourselves to do some things rather than others. Motivation isn't constant. It dips and wanes and even disappears at times, so we need to be prepared to find ways to self-motivate.

Where does motivation come from?

Motivation comes from internal or external sources – it can be intrinsic or extrinsic.

Intrinsic motivation is a drive that comes from within. It is a powerful motivator as it is inextricably tied up with your sense of identity. For example, people who are intrinsically motivated to play sport do so because they love playing the sport itself, and so it forms part of their identity.

I love training with a team as I feel a sense of purpose, commitment and challenge. Training sessions – despite being physically tough at times – were commitments in my week that I looked forward to (except for the fitness tests!). I loved focusing on improving my skills, through setting individual milestones and goals. I always felt hugely grateful to be part of the team, but as an individual it was important to me that I contributed to and enhanced the collective. That always drove me on.

Extrinsic motivation is driven by external reward. We might do it for praise and recognition from others, or for tangible reward, and often for both. Take doing our jobs as an example. Many of us are motivated to do it for tangible, monetary gain, i.e. to get a wage. Some people will also be intrinsically motivated to do their job because they are passionate about it and want to succeed.

I remember the first day of filming the RTÉ documentary series *Why Girls Quit Sport*. I had to address a school assembly packed with teenage girls, ranging from twelve to eighteen years old. What a daunting prospect. Teenagers can be an intimidating bunch. I had to go into a school in inner-city Dublin and appeal to them to take part in the show. I was essentially trying to entice girls who had never played sport, or had once played but dropped out, to sign up to my sports team. I knew getting buy-in could prove challenging.

On the morning of the assembly, I remember sitting in my car outside the school, and I was so nervous I had to give myself a pep talk for twenty minutes before finally plucking up the courage to go inside. I had to remind myself that this was important to me, that I was capable of dealing with any questions they fired at me and any obstacles I faced. In their eyes, I could have been just a Cork culchie, so I really felt the pressure to win these girls over. Ultimately, I needed to motivate myself first, so I could motivate them to get involved.

The key principles of motivation

We all know that just because we want to achieve something doesn't mean we will achieve it. We must be able to actively pursue our goal, persist through obstacles and have the endurance to complete the journey. There are three main tenets of motivation: targeting, perseverance and intensity.

- **Targeting** – this is the decision to set goals and ensure that they are monitored on a regular basis.
- **Perseverance** – this is the continued effort towards a goal, even though you encounter obstacles.
- **Intensity** – this is the amount of energy and effort that you devote to the activity. What is your level of commitment?

These three principles are symbiotic – all three need to be in play for you to stay motivated. However, it is the degree to which you engage each individual component that can impact on whether you achieve your goal. If you have strong targets, you are likely to make a good start pursuing the goal, but if you lack perseverance and intensity, it is unlikely you will succeed in achieving it.

Reframing goals helps with motivation

Motivating ourselves can be difficult. Flipping the narrative from negative to positive can help. Take exercise, for example. We often view exercise as a chore, something unenjoyable. Why is it that when the bell goes for break time in primary school, children run out with smiling faces and then run around for half an hour, and they look forward all week to their PE classes on a Friday afternoon? The idea of exercise may have been distorted in the minds of adults, but it hasn't happened in children . . . at least, not yet.

Based on countless conversations I have had, exercise is

something many people feel they *must* do to have something else that they consider a reward. But what if exercise is its own reward and we just can't see it? What if – just like time on the couch, or a hot bath, or a meal out – exercise is something we can enjoy doing AND reap the benefits from? We need to flip the narrative from 'I've *got* to do this' to 'I *get* to do this'.

Those of us who can exercise are privileged to do so. Many are incapacitated, injured or ill and would love the opportunity. Those of us who can should embrace it, while we are able to. This is your reminder that exercise is not meant to be a punishment for when you overindulge. It doesn't exist for the sole purpose of weight loss, even though this may be the reality for those who have a negative relationship with exercise, because they associate it with wanting to shed pounds. It is so much harder to motivate yourself to do something when you think about it in a negative way.

Tips for staying motivated

If the initial fire and drive that you had when you started the journey to your goal has dampened down slightly, it is possible to find that spark and get motivated again.

- **Adjust your goals** – goals do not need to be fixed
  and immovable ideals. Sometimes we change
  during the process, and this may mean that we

need to adjust our goals slightly to make them more meaningful to us at any given time. The more important something is to you, the more likely it is that you'll be motivated to achieve it.

- **Review your goals** – check if they are realistic in the time frame you have set. Sometimes a goal can be so huge and overwhelming that we just feel like a failure if it's not immediately attainable. In the previous chapter I touched on the idea of incorporating a series of milestones to target along the way. Break down your goal into a series of milestones and you'll be amazed at how much more motivated you'll be.

- **Remind yourself about how far you've already come** – think about what you've achieved and give credit to your strengths.

- **Maintain momentum** – research conducted by University College London has shown that it takes sixty-six days on average to form a new habit from the first time the new action is undertaken (contrary to the common myth that it's twenty-one days). Keeping a routine is the best way of keeping up momentum.

- **Surround yourself with a positive support system** – this might seem straightforward, but many of us welcome toxic people into our lives. You know, the ones who pass judgement instead of wholeheartedly supporting us. It's hard to stay motivated when others force you to doubt yourself.

Take a moment to appreciate the view!

Think about climbing up a mountain. Most of us would have aspirations to reach the summit. Suddenly, just when you think you are at the top, you realize it's a fake summit and you still have quite a way to go. You feel demotivated, demoralized and downhearted!

Stop! Pause and take a moment and turn around so you can look down to where you first started. I guarantee, you will be surprised at just how far you have climbed. Take in the view. Let that motivate you to push forward. You have reached that point by simply putting one foot in front of the other. We all need to take the time to acknowledge the effort required in getting to where we are right now. We mightn't be anywhere near the top yet, but we are further along than we often realize.

Motivating others

We are incredibly complex beings. We all interpret things in different ways based on previous experiences and beliefs, so when trying to motivate others, we need to be aware that everyone comes from a different place. At the heart of motivating others is connection. There must be trust, under-standing and respect to motivate successfully.

Stephen R. Covey writes in his book *The 7 Habits of Highly Effective People* that we should 'seek first to understand then to be understood' (Habit 5). This means that you must be willing to listen to other people, to their viewpoints, to their way of doing things, to their ideas. At times, you may need to adapt your style to effectively connect with them.

I love to talk, as anyone who knows me will confirm. I've made a career out of it. From my experience in various roles as a captain of sports teams, as a broadcaster interviewing people or as a coach on *Ireland's Fittest Family*, I've had to learn and practise active listening with others. I've realized that you'll never be able to connect with, motivate or inspire others to action if you're the one talking all the time.

As a coach on *Ireland's Fittest Family*, I quickly learned the valuable lesson that motivation is a key component of the show. While the viewers might see the coaches getting animated during the races, what they may not see is the quieter moments of motivation with individual family members. When you are motivating others, you need to know what makes them tick, how to speak to them, what language to use. Trust is established in these exchanges.

When you are motivating others, particularly in a competi-tive context, some people want you to strongly encourage them and hold them accountable, while others need a gentler approach. If you watch the famous Hang Tough challenge, you may notice that sometimes I am more vocal with certain family members, getting on their case, almost applying pressure. With others, I am calmer and more relaxed. As a sportsperson, I liked pressure being applied – it made me perform better. But a vital part of motivating others is understanding that what works for you may not work for others and you have to adapt your strategies accordingly.

10. Tactics board for purpose

'The greatest thing in this world is not so much where
we stand as in what direction we are moving'
– Johann Wolfgang von Goethe

As we move and evolve through our lives, we find ourselves juggling with so much. The intensity of balancing family, finances, careers and relationships can sometimes cause us to lose sense of what makes us feel fulfilled. It's time to take charge of our own sense of contentment by working out what we want from life, and what our purpose is. Ask yourself what is important in your life. Where do you get your energy from? What makes you get out of bed in the morning?

Little pockets of joy fuel me. When I experience joy, I feel re-energized. Exercise is a provider of said joy. It's different for everyone. Some people find their joy in journalling, or from sitting in the garden with a coffee, or going for a run. Find out what yours is. Work out your values and get in tune with what you want out of life. You will feel more fulfilled, and the time you invest in yourself is never going to be wasted. We need time to eat better, to exercise more, to spend time with the people we love, and it is equally important to find the time for investing in what makes our souls happy.

Anna's take-home points

- **Identify your *purpose*** – what is your 'why' in life? Living with a purposeful approach to life makes you feel more in control of your future and improves your mental health.
- **Determine your *values*** – what are the values that you want to live your life by? Aligning your values with your purpose will help you discover what you want out of life and set you on the course to achieving it.
- **Set *goals*** – identify what you can do in daily life that will help you achieve your sense of purpose. Don't be afraid to adjust the goalposts.
- **Keep your *future self* in mind** – remember that every decision you make today affects who you become tomorrow.
- **Practise *motivation*** – you will have great days and you will have not-so-great days. Find out what keeps you motivated and use it.

Read

Start With Why – Simon Sinek
The 7 Habits of Highly Effective People – Stephen R. Covey
Be Your Future Self Now – Dr Benjamin Hardy

The 4–7 Zone – Dr Colman Noctor
The Daily Stoic – Ryan Holiday
101 Essays That Will Change the Way You Think – Brianna
Wiest

Listen

Power Hour podcast– Adrienne Herbert
Where is My Mind? podcast – Niall Breslin
'Never Forget' – Take That
'Starlight' – Westlife
'Dreams' – The Cranberries

Watch

Coach Carter
Field of Dreams
Gladiator
Break Point
Remember the Titans

Notes

Purpose – my personal tactics board

....

....

....

....

....

....

....

....

....

....

....

....

PART THREE

Game Plan for Consistency

11. Consistency can change your life

'Success isn't always about greatness.
It's about consistency. Consistent hard
work leads to success. Greatness will come'
— Dwayne Johnson

Playing camogie from such an early age has taught me so many life lessons. There were ten girls in my Junior Infants class at Milford National School, and plenty more in the classes ahead. We all started playing together in school and with our newly formed camogie club. We were successful quite quickly, winning tournaments like the Community Games in Mosney (who remembers Mosney?!) and the GAA's primary schools' organization in Cork, Sciath na Scol.

By the time I got into St Mary's Secondary School, Charleville, I had already experienced a considerable amount of sporting success for a twelve-year-old. So, of course, when the trials happened for the school camogie team, I enthusiastically tried out.

I vividly remember all the girls huddled around the noticeboard in the canteen checking to see who had made the squads. There was a Junior A and a B squad. Much to my huge dismay, I didn't make the A team. That really stung. I was named on the Junior B team, and I could only watch on as my primary school teammates played for the school in tournaments for the Junior As. It certainly was a blow to my confidence (which wasn't exactly operating at a high level as it was).

The realization that I wasn't as good as many of my Milford teammates in the eyes of the school manager was so tough to take. I think I had a few tantrums at home, but then after one tantrum too many, my dad turned around and said to me, 'Okay, so now what are you going to do about it?' It lit something within me. There *were* things I could do. So, I kept going, I consistently went to training, showed up and did my best, and always tried to work hard.

The truth was that I loved the game, it was – at that time – such a big part of who I was, and I wanted to be one of the best. And then, halfway through the year, the manager called me into his classroom and informed me that he wanted me to bring my gear to the Junior A Munster Final that weekend.

It was like Christmas had come early. I was so excited even though I knew I was going as a sub, but it was more about what it represented to me. He was acknowledging my effort, my improvement at training, my dedication, my progress, my consistency. I sat on the bench for most of the match, and towards the end I was brought on. I gave the match everything I had. I played with the Junior A team for the rest of the year. By second year, I was playing on the Senior A team.

What had changed in that twelve months? I had learned that developing a strong work ethic was within my control when so much else wasn't. I came across a quote back then that stuck with me: 'Hard work will beat talent when talent doesn't work hard.' Also, up until secondary school, while I was undoubtedly determined, I had so often let my fear of making mistakes on the pitch hold me back. It stifled my playing ability and my confidence.

Mr Harrington, our manager, encouraged us to remove the focus from the mistakes and focus instead on the recovery. He instilled in us that when you lost the ball you worked twice as hard to get it back. That was what mattered most. As a result of his patience and approach, when I lost the ball he would gently remind me to go again, reinforcing the emphasis on work ethic. I was more determined than ever to try harder. The environment created around our school team nurtured my love of the game even more. It also cleverly disguised the learning curve, which was to have the courage to try, to just go for it, while training extremely hard.

And things progressed from there – by age twelve, having transitioned to the Junior A team, I was also playing on the Cork Under-16 team. By thirteen, I was playing on the Cork Under-18 team. And by sixteen, I was on the Cork Senior panel. Any trophies and titles I won as part of subsequent teams all came from that secret to success I learned in the first year of secondary school.

I don't think it was a coincidence that during my six years at St Mary's we won ten All-Ireland school titles. We had talent for sure, but it was the environment and culture fostered by the coaches that allowed us to flourish. I now had in my arsenal the skill to recover quickly from a mistake, along with the determination and drive to rectify it. And that skill has served me throughout my life, not just on the playing field.

Habits are the key to consistency

The concept of consistency has been drilled into me from an early age, and I credit it with the successes I have had on and off the pitch. To me, consistency means focusing on the task at hand in the present moment, knowing that it feeds into your long-term goals. To be consistent, we need to see the value in what we are doing. This all ties in with developing a strong sense of purpose with regards to your goals. To make any sustainable lifestyle change, the most important factor in its success is consistency.

I will talk about creating new, positive habits in chapter 13. By relying on new habits that correlate with your goals, you will free up your mental energy to reach your full potential. I will also talk about the value of commitment, as commitment is the key to consistency. Once we make a commitment to do something, we will consistently try to achieve it. It's not the big changes, not the dramatic overhauls, that can transform your life. It's the small, incremental changes repeated time and time again that make the biggest difference. As the famous quote attributed to Aristotle goes, 'We are what we repeatedly do. Excellence, then, is not an act, but a habit.'

Consistency is about showing up every day for YOU in different aspects of your life. Do five minutes, honour that commitment, allow space in your day. Just start – it's the hardest bit to do.

When it comes to consistency, imagine the goal to be a house under construction, and the habits and processes are the scaffolding. If you don't have stable supports, your house, your goal, will collapse.

12. The promise of commitment

'Things never happen on accident. They happen
because you have a vision, you have a commitment,
you have a dream'
— Oscar de la Renta

Commitment is essentially a promise to do something. When we make a promise to achieve a certain outcome, we must also be willing to undertake the process that is necessary to achieve this outcome. Commitment is one of the most important skills you can learn – and I say learn, as it is a skill that needs to be worked on to improve. People underestimate the value of sport, but you must commit to turning up to training and matches, or you let yourself and your teammates down. They are relying on you. On a deeper level, *you* are relying on you, and if you commit to something, you must be willing to do it.

Pursuing a goal takes courage, but it also takes a lot of work and discipline. I believe commitment is a silent pact that you make with yourself when you are chasing a goal, a target or a dream. Commitment is doing what you said you would do, even when you don't want to do it. It starts and ends with you. The good news is that commitment is a characteristic that can be developed. It's like a muscle – the more you invest in building it up, the stronger it gets.

Keeping a commitment to yourself is the first step you must take in achieving any goal. It's a skill that needs to be practised. Stay with me on this . . . if you just commit to turning up for a run in the morning, everything else will fall into place after that. Let me break it down.

Turning up for the run is the commitment. You don't have a commitment to any of the details, only to the act of showing up. It's irrelevant what time you complete the run in, or how far you run, or what your running technique is like. Your commitment is in the fact that you turn up to do it. Just to run.

If you turn up, even if you don't run fast or for long, you will feel you have honoured that commitment to yourself. You kept your promise to yourself. That's where your self-belief and confidence develops, in knowing you are capable and disciplined enough to keep a commitment.

I believe that commitment is strongly connected to consistency. Consistency is about showing up in some capacity on a regular basis, contributing towards something regardless of mood, emotions or circumstance. We may have committed to showing up for the first run, but one run isn't going to get us to our goal. We must commit consistently.

We have been programmed to think that we must be able to dedicate 100 per cent to our goals all the time, but that is not realistic. We have to accept that sometimes life can get in the way, but if your commitment to your goal is strong enough, you will find a way to do *something*.

Showing up daily

What we think it means:

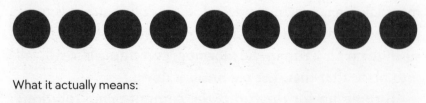

What it actually means:

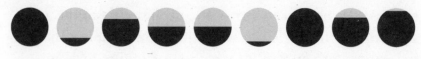

To take the running example, say things are going great the first few mornings, then on the fourth day you wake up and it's raining. You are lying in bed telling yourself you can't go. You *want* to go, but it's the weather's fault. Or you stayed up late the night before and when your alarm goes off you pull the blankets over your head and blame Netflix for giving you the opportunity to watch the next episode on demand. So, you have a choice: stay in bed or commit to your goal. What, then, has a major bearing on that choice? Your level of commitment to that goal.

Why have you decided to get up every morning to go for a run? Why is it important to you? For your physical health? For your headspace? Because it makes you feel better? Analysing why you are doing something is crucial to your ability to commit to it. Then being consistent with it will mean that

144

you show up. Even if it's only for a fifteen-minute jog instead of a thirty-minute run.

> **'You are what you do,
> not what you say you'll do' – Carl Jung**
>
> Commitment is doing what you said you would do, even when you don't want to do it. So, doing the thing you committed to doing becomes a part of your self-identity.
>
> For instance, for me a simple daily commitment is to put on my exercise gear first thing in the morning. Even when I'm not in the mood to exercise, and I just want to go back to bed, I will put it on. Once it's on, that's the hardest part done. And more often than not, I will honour my commitment to myself and do some form of movement. Then the endorphins and feel-good factor will follow – not just because of the exercise but because I am doing something that aligns with who I want to be and how I want to see myself.

In chapter 8 we learned how to set out our goals. We know what we want to achieve, and we have the motivation to do it. How do we stay committed to achieving these goals?

Make an action plan

Write out an action plan that details each step you need to take to achieve your goal. Plan your route. Each step builds on the last, bringing you closer to the finishing line.

1. **Focus on one goal** – Put your energy into achieving one goal. If you try to do too much at once, you could find it overwhelming and set yourself up for failure.

2. **Research, research, research** – Carry out as much research as possible. Read relevant blogs and articles, listen to podcasts, talk to people who have achieved that particular goal before. These sources can help you work out the necessary steps for hitting your target.

3. **Have a clear timeline and deadline** – You need to set out clear time frames for each milestone along the way. Have a defined deadline in place to keep you motivated.

4. **Track your progress** – Print out your action plan and put it somewhere visible or have it easily accessible on your phone. Each time you hit a milestone, tick it off. Seeing the proof of your achievements will motivate you to keep going.

146

5. **Reward yourself!** – It's important to reward yourself when you hit each milestone. Use it to incentivize you.

The 1 per cent improvements

Focusing on the 1 per cent improvements is one of my core principles when it comes to progressing towards goals. We often strive for perfection when it comes to getting healthier and fitter, or around any other goal we have. If we can't do it perfectly, then we can be guilty of adopting the attitude 'Why bother?' I believe we need to turn our attention to striving for progress.

Let's break down your day: there are twenty-four hours in your day, which is 1,440 minutes. If you take 1 per cent of that, it equates to approximately fifteen minutes. If you dedicated just 1 per cent of each day to reaching your goal, in a year that's over ninety hours you have invested in achieving your goal! Imagine what you could do with ninety hours! It can be achieved with a little commitment.

If you feel you don't know where to start, just focus on achieving 1 per cent. All of those 1 per cents will then accumulate over time. Block out time in your schedule for today's 1 per cent and make it happen. Then do the same tomorrow and so forth.

The key is being consistent with that 1 per cent.

Commit to commitment

'Commitment is an act, not a word'
— Jean-Paul Sartre

A lot of us define success by reaching the end goal, whatever that may be for us. We rarely acknowledge the countless hours that have been poured into the *process* of trying to get there. Why is that? Why do we not celebrate our willingness to commit to something, even if we don't come out on top?

Unfortunately, many of us are conditioned to think that it's only the bottom line which matters. That unless we achieve the goal, then everything up until that point is almost rendered meaningless. In sport, there will only ever be one winner, so if you define your success only by whether you come first, then you will rarely experience the feeling of success.

We tell children that, no matter what happens, it's the taking part that counts. But do we truly believe that for ourselves? If a child is learning to ride a bike, and falls off a hundred times, we encourage them to get back on for the 101st time. We remind them to keep trying and we praise them for that. Yet, as adults, the narrative changes. We demand the best from ourselves continuously, both publicly and privately. We berate ourselves if we come up short. The act of trying is ignored in favour of the attainment of excellence.

Commitment and winning are not mutually exclusive. In fact, committing to something does not guarantee results, but without commitment any attempts are futile.

Five ways to commit to commitment

1. Time slot

You should set yourself a specific time slot when you are going to do your task each day and stick to it as much as possible. It is much easier to commit knowing that time dedicated to your goal is blocked out each day. Your mind is also more likely to adapt and accept it, as the brain loves routine.

Top tip: we schedule our work meetings and our children's extra-curricular activities into our diaries. Do the same with your own personal priorities, whether they are exercise-related, fun-related, etc. A handy way to identify which category they fall into is to highlight them in different colours on your calendar. Work is blue, Family is green, Exercise is yellow, Fun is red, etc. Then, if you don't see a colour featuring much in your diary, you know you need to schedule more of it in.

This provides a great visual representation for life activities and helps with accountability.

2. Morning bird or night owl?

Take time to identify when you are at your 'peak'. Are you more alert in the mornings or evenings? Do you love getting up early each day, or do you come to life at night? It's not just about when you have free time, it's as important to understand when you have the most energy and concentration. This will allow you to better sustain your commitment levels when it comes to your goals.

3. Reasons versus excuses

Distinguish between reasons and excuses to help you stay committed. Life situations can sometimes prevent us from following through on what we said we would do. There is no denying that, but when does a reason become an excuse? An excuse is a justification or way to defend an action. We can tell ourselves that we had no control over the outcome, therefore no fault rests with us. Reasons become excuses when they are consciously used to avoid responsibility. Usually when you have a valid reason for not doing something, you will find another way, even if it is at a deferred time.

Let's go back to the earlier running example. Say you have committed to getting up before work to exercise. You have planned to go for an early-morning run and when you wake up it is raining, so you tell yourself you can't go. If you don't go, that is simply an excuse that you're making for yourself. You can easily overcome the obstacle by simply wearing a raincoat. However, say your child is sick and needs care so you cannot leave them – that is a legitimate reason. Perhaps you can find an alternative time and go for the run on your lunch break or after work instead. Or even turn a work call into a 'walk and talk' call as an alternative.

4. Identify obstacles

When you are committing to anything, identify in advance the potential obstacles that might challenge said commitment. Once you identify the potential stumbling blocks, you can come up with ways to counteract them. There are always going to be unforeseen things that blindside you, but if you are prepared for the most part, you will find it easier to preserve your commitment levels.

For example, say you are trying to eat healthier, but you know that traffic might cause you to get delayed coming home from work. By batch cooking for the next day, you won't have to worry about cooking if you get home late.

5. Back-up plan

Commit to your plan of action. Sometimes thing don't go as planned, and when things go unexpectedly wrong it can be debilitating and uncomfortable. The simple truth is that this is a regular occurrence in life, so we need to get comfortable with the uncomfortable. We need to be able to adapt. Anyone having a baby will tell you this. You can have your birthing plan perfected, but the reality of the situation means that this can change in an instant!

Visualizing alternatives can help if you need to deviate unexpectedly. When I was playing camogie, I used visualization techniques regularly to envision different scenarios. Sure, I had a plan for how I wanted things to pan out, a strategy for how I was going to beat my opponent, but I would also have to think 'What happens if I fall as I race to the ball?' 'What will I do if the opposing player gets past me?' If it did happen, I felt like I was somewhat prepared for the consequences.

I would recommend creating a back-up plan to have as a fall-back when something unexpected happens. For example, you have a plan centred about getting fitter and you intend to go to the gym on the way to work, but the road to the gym is closed off so you can't go. Having a pair of runners and a coat in your car as a back-up means you can still exercise and keep yourself on track in some capacity, so you maintain your commitment to your fitness goal.

The importance of committing when the unexpected happens

Legendary swimmer Michael Phelps is the holder of twenty-eight Olympic medals, twenty-three of them gold, so he knows a thing or two about preparation and commitment. He used to spend hours visualizing a race. He thought about how he wanted it to go, how he didn't want it to go and how it could go. Having a plan for the bad moments was just as important to him so that he didn't panic if he was faced with an unexpected situation.

During the 200m butterfly final at the 2008 Beijing Olympics, his goggles filled up with water, forcing him to swim blind for most of the race. Not only did he still go on to win the gold medal, he set a new world record. Afterwards, he spoke about how he had visualized in training what he would do if his goggles ever did fill with water. He used to count his strokes while doing lengths of the pool in case he couldn't see, and when it happened, he simply reverted to counting his strokes, allowing him to time his turn at the wall perfectly and not lose momentum.

Don't give in to negativity or doubt

So, you're committed to achieving your goal, but what happens when you hit the inevitable stumbling block along the way? And it is inevitable that you will because no path to success runs smoothly. We have already discussed negative self-talk in chapter 2 and it is in these scenarios where we have to reframe the negative into a positive. We need to empower ourselves to push forward, and I have fully embraced a concept called 'the power of not yet', pioneered by Stanford professor Carol Dweck, when times get a little tough.

The power of not yet

Saying 'I can't do X' is a prime example of a self-limiting belief. This is an assumption or a perception that you have about yourself and about the way the world works. These assumptions are called self-limiting because in some way they are holding you back from seeing yourself as the person you can be, and from achieving what you are truly capable of in life. But you know what? It's just a story you're telling yourself and you need to replace this belief with something that empowers you instead. If you keep telling yourself that you're not good enough, then you will eventually start to believe it.

As Henry Ford said, 'Whether you think you can, or you think you can't – you're right.'

The language we use when we are speaking to ourselves

plays a big part in overturning our self-limiting beliefs. They may be words we never say aloud, but if we are saying them internally, they still carry huge weight.

Our language selection can change the meaning of a statement:

I can't do it . . . yet.

I'm not fit enough . . . yet.

I'm not knowledgeable enough . . . yet.

Within these statements is the acknowledgement that we have the power to change the outcome.

The correct use of language helps reframe and retrain our mindset and transforms it from self-limiting to self-empowering. I use the word 'empowering' here instead of 'positive' because the word 'positive' is misinterpreted. We don't always need to be positive; sometimes we can feel negatively towards something and still be empowered by it.

Saying something like 'I'm not fit enough for a 10km run yet' is empowering, because it gives you a target and a goal and moves you towards it. Even if you never make it, that little tweak using the word 'yet' may just change how you feel towards it. You maintain your commitment and your motivation to keep going until you hit it. It allows you to embrace consistency in your commitment and, day by day, step by step, you will make it.

The W.I.N. system

Bob Bowman was Michael Phelps's swim coach for over twenty years, and he implemented a system he called the W.I.N. system. W.I.N. stands for 'What's important now?'

You see, when you commit to something, it's common that after a short time something will get in the way, and often – given the way we are all told to be in touch with our emotions – we think we are putting ourselves first by listening to our feelings or listening to our bodies. The trouble with that is that emotions are not a good judge of what we need or what we should do.

Bowman's idea was that instead of asking yourself what you want or how you feel, ask yourself 'What's important now?' By asking this we can get closer to what we really want and stay committed to the goal. Feelings can lead us astray, and what we need to know in these situations is where we are going and why. By asking ourselves that question, we can show up for ourselves even when we don't want to.

Have a strong support system

Having people who support you along the way is invaluable. They keep you in check and help keep you motivated and committed to your goals. Join a running club, or a regular gym class, or a reading group. Your family and friends can also give you positive reinforcement and constructive advice when you need it.

While it is important to keep your distance from negative and defeatist people, you still need people who keep you grounded and give you the facts. Encouragement isn't always about giving compliments and pats on the back. A support system needs an open and honest channel of communication. It's about telling you what you need to hear too, even when you don't want to hear it, but only with the aim of helping you.

My parents have always been my biggest support system – they were always there, on the good and the bad days, and were great at keeping me grounded, my dad in particular!

Back in September 2010, I got my first taste of live broadcasting as I was asked to co-commentate on RTÉ Radio 1 with the GAA legend Mícheál Ó Muircheartaigh. Cork had contested every Senior Camogie All-Ireland Final since I had joined the panel in 2003, but that year we had lost in the All-Ireland Semi-Final after a replay. It was bittersweet to be asked to co-commentate, because I yearned to be out there playing, but it was my first time on RTÉ Radio 1 and who better to make my debut with than an RTÉ icon? Mícheál was the voice of the GAA, a huge figure in Irish sport, so it was such an honour to sit in the crow's nest in Croke Park with him and commentate on the Final.

The next day I sought out my dad, knowing he would have been listening intently. I was a little smug about my endeavours. I was young and excited from the momentous day. I found Dad reading the newspaper in the kitchen and I asked him for the breakdown, the specifics, how I did, how I sounded, what I said. I obviously wanted to hear all good things.

'So, you didn't hear about Mícheál Ó Muircheartaigh?' Dad replied coolly.

I shook my head. 'What about him?'

'He announced his retirement today,' Dad replied, raising an eyebrow and observing my face for my reaction. By now I was even more smug, thinking that I was one of the last to ever commentate with this great man. My dad continued to concentrate on reading the paper, so I couldn't see the mischief in his eyes or his wry smile developing. 'Imagine, that man gave decades to Irish sports broadcasting,' he said, 'and one hour with you and he decides to call it a day.'

I was highly indignant at the time, of course, but that was my dad's 'affectionate' way of keeping me grounded, keeping me focused and keeping me committed to pushing ahead. He was always straight-talking with me (even when I didn't want to hear it), always pointing out ways to help me improve on the pitch. He saw it as his role to keep my ego in check. At home, my head never stayed in the clouds for long because, while my parents loved to see me do well, they also knew the importance of being realistic, striving to improve in all aspects of life, and – in typical Irish fashion – they never let me get too far ahead of myself.

Trains and drains!

There are generally two types of people in your life – energy trains and energy drains. The trains can be described as the steam engines in your life. They are full of encouragement and positive support, driving you on to achieve better things. The drains are exactly what the name suggests – they drain your energy. They are the ones who are always finding things to complain about: 'Ugh, I can't believe it's only Tuesday, the weekend is aaaages away!' 'Can you believe she wants me to do this?' 'How come she got that and I didn't?' They are the ones who tend to drag you down when you are trying to make a positive change in your life: 'Why aren't you drinking? You're so boring!' 'Why bother going for that walk at lunchtime, come for a pizza with us.'

Do they make you feel better in their company? How is your energy after spending time with both types of person? Do you recognize these types of people in your family/friendship groups/colleague circle?

Research suggests we are the product of the five people we spend the most time with, so pick your team carefully. When you are committed to achieving your goal, surround yourself with the ones you know will support and not discourage you.

Remember, persistence beats resistance. What we do for ourselves today will stand to us down the line, even if we are only taking baby steps.

13. Our brains love routine

'Success is the sum of small efforts
repeated day in and day out'
— Robert Collier

It is vital that you plan ahead and do the things today that will help you in the future. I saw a poster in my gym recently that reaffirmed this for me: 'Excuses make today easier, but tomorrow harder – discipline makes today harder, but tomorrow easier.'

How can we create discipline in our lives and ensure we remain committed to our goals? Habits and routines are the answer.

A lot of us already have a daily routine fixed into place. The alarm goes off and we begin our morning routine of getting ready for the day ahead. Routines are a normal part of life for everyone. You see, the human brain loves things to stay the same. It prefers us to do what we already know, so it doesn't expend energy learning and storing new information. It's always easier to stay where we are and do what we know how to do, and the brain wants our life like that. It prefers familiar things.

There are lots of positives to routines. Research shows that routine creates structure and plays an important part in improving mental, emotional and physical health. A good routine will lower cortisol levels, which is great for stress management. Routines encourage self-care; they lift your mood and can enhance your focus. Routines also help with time management, which leads to feelings of accomplishment.

The absence of routine can often lead to feelings of unmanageability or a lack of control. The human brain loves to know what it's doing and resists change for this reason, as when things are familiar, cortisol levels don't spike as often and you feel less stress.

Think about times when you've started a new job or a new course and you've come home feeling exhausted, even though you were sitting down the whole time. It's because the brain uses real energy in new environments. It's why travel to new places can be tiring, because you need to think and work things out as you go along. An hour on the plane feels more draining than an hour in the car to work, because it's all new information and out of our normal routine.

Sometimes, to commit to achieving a new goal, we need to switch up our routine and form new habits. Think about this when you start to struggle, or when you feel like you can't commit: your brain is actively working against you. Your brain doesn't want to take notes. This is due to what's called 'homeostasis'. Homeostasis relates to maintaining equilibrium. Our brains and bodies, and even our behaviours, have an in-built tendency to want to stay the same, to remain within certain limits, and therefore will want to revert to what is familiar when we attempt to change things.

This default desire to maintain the status quo is why you

may find yourself slipping back into your assigned 'role' in certain life situations – the role you play within your family, in your friendship circle, at work, in a relationship or on a team, even if it's a role you don't necessarily want to fulfil. We often give ourselves a hard time when this happens: 'I promised myself I'd stop doing that. Why did I do it again?' Does this sound familiar? You can stop beating yourself up as making change challenges your brain, whereas sticking to your familiar role removes the complexity of having to figure things out. I will talk lots more about roles in the next chapter.

Every one of us resists significant change to varying degrees, even change for the better. At the start of anything new, your brain has to use a lot of energy just processing and working things out. Take a new job as an example. The first few days your brain is tired, learning new systems and instructions. If you commit and persevere, and get familiar with whatever the new activity is, you will notice the time it takes to do it shortens, and your brain stops seeing the activity as new and as something to be resisted. As we discussed earlier, motivation can dip and wain, and as James Clear says in his book *Atomic Habits*, 'You do not rise to the level of your goals. You fall to the level of your systems [habits],' so you need to make sure your habits are serving you.

How to build a new routine

First, we must differentiate between a habit and a routine. A routine is a series of behaviours that are frequently repeated, with intention and conscious effort, like doing the laundry every day. A habit is something we do with little or no conscious thought, like washing our hands or grabbing a couple of biscuits if we're feeling tired or stressed. Our brain goes on to autopilot mode. We'll first look at building a new routine, and then we'll look at the new habits we can incorporate into the routine. With these two working together cohesively, you should be able to make some positive changes.

If we always have the same routines, we can start to feel 'stuck' or bored in our lives, so learning to adapt and add to our routines is necessary for growth and personal development. The challenge is to pace ourselves, as drastic changes in routine rarely continue into the longer term, so they need to be gradual.

One way to uncover your current routines is to make a list of what you do daily, Monday to Sunday – things that never change. Maybe you always start your day with coffee, maybe you have a shower first, maybe you walk the dog. Take a sheet of paper and make three columns – headed 'Morning', 'Afternoon' and 'Evening' – and under each heading list the basic must-dos of your day.

When you look at your lists, you may see some patterns. For instance, your current morning routine may be to wake up at 7.30 a.m. to optimize the amount of time you spend in bed. So, you wake up and rush into the shower, get ready and head into work, skipping breakfast. By 11 a.m. you are starving and head to the café to pick up a muffin and a latte.

Coming up with the best plan for Team Me

So that we can consciously design routines that work for us, we need to identify our goals and spend time thinking about what we are aiming to achieve in the short-, medium- and long-term.

We also need to consider the things that support living well:

- Being physically active
- Rest, recovery and quality sleep
- Carving out time to do things you love
- Eating regular balanced meals
- Having realistic, attainable goals
- Challenging yourself
- Consistent contact with loved ones
- Finding joy and adopting optimism

How can we incorporate all these into our daily routines? What do we need to change and what can stay the same?

Remember, you are the captain of Team Me. Put yourself in charge of your routine and you will find that it can be really rewarding and can help you maintain a sense of control in life. Focus on what you have control of and adjust your routines to match that. Sticking to a basic structure for eating, sleeping and exercise helps you feel able to make other decisions throughout the day. Slotting in certain reliable routines can optimize time, mood and energy levels. They can allow you to keep committed to your goals.

So, taking the example above – of staying in bed till the last possible moment, skipping breakfast and then grabbing a mid-morning muffin – how about you wake up at 7.15 a.m. and give yourself time after you get ready to have a quick healthy breakfast? Maybe some overnight oats you prepared the night before or a couple of boiled eggs. You feel full, satisfied and energetic going into work and over time your 11 a.m. cravings disappear.

Change your habits

'We all deal with setbacks but in the long run, the quality of our lives often depends on the quality of our habits. With the same habits, you'll end up with the same results. But with better habits, anything is possible'
— James Clear

As I mentioned above, habits are the small daily decisions you make and the actions you perform which become automatic, unconscious and reoccurring behaviours. When I was trying to break some bad habits I found James Clear's book *Atomic Habits* helpful in allowing me to understand the psychology behind habit-forming and how to change them for the better. He believes that making one small change to your habits over time will have a cumulative effect and lead to significant results, not to mention a sense of control over your life.

When I am trying to build new habits, I find it is easier to add something in than to cut something out. If you want to eat healthier meals, don't try to eliminate certain foods, instead add in extra portions of food that will nourish you.

James Clear identified the stages of habit formation as the **cue**, the **craving**, the **response** and the **reward**, and every single habit we have is linked to these four stages:

1. The **cue** triggers the brain to notice an opportunity for a reward or pleasure. A cue can be a smell, a sound, an event, an interaction, or anything else that then triggers a desire. This desire is known as the craving.

2. The **craving** is an internal, emotional response attached to a particular cue. That craving then motivates you or prompts you to act.

3. The **response** is the actual behaviour, or habit, performed to obtain the change you desire. Your brain prompts you to take a certain action it believes will create the feeling of satisfaction you want.

4. The **reward** is the satisfaction gained from the action taken. The brain builds a pathway from the cue to this state of pleasure. Every time you experience the same cue, the brain will be triggered to desire that pleasure again. You will be prompted to perform the same action, thereby creating a habit.

The more you repeat a habit, the more you will go through these stages without even thinking about them. It becomes an automatic behaviour. An example of the habit process would work like this:

1. The **cue** – you walk past a coffee shop on the way to work and smell freshly roasted coffee.

2. The **craving** – coffee gives you energy, and you want to feel energized.

3. The **response** – you buy a cup of coffee.

4. The **reward** – by the time you reach work, you are raring to go. Buying a cup of coffee becomes associated with your walk to work.

It's fascinating when you begin to understand how a habit is formed, and it explains why we do what we do. Habits can take over as a form of automated solution in our everyday lives, created as our brains understand our repeated behaviours. As a result of putting these in place, our brains can conserve energy and are freed up to focus on ad hoc things that crop up, like problem-solving.

An important takeaway for me is knowing that our cues start the whole process off, therefore we need to become more aware of the potential cues in our lives that may set habits in motion: the smell of fresh bread in a shop, the ding of a WhatsApp notification, the box of sweets left open on the counter.

Training your brain into forming good habits

One thing to note when it comes to habits is that your brain doesn't identify if a habit is helping or hindering you. It cannot differentiate between 'good' and 'bad' habits, it just identifies the reoccurring behaviours in our lives and begins to form the habits.

How do we replace bad habits with good habits? Clear suggests that we use his 'Four Laws of Behaviour Change' to establish new habits.

So, to form good habits:

1. The **cue** – make it obvious.

2. The **craving** – make it attractive.

3. The **response** – make it easy.

4. The **reward** – make it satisfying.

For example:

1. The **cue** – I place my exercise gear beside my bed so it is ready to put on straight away in the morning i.e. make it obvious.

2. The **craving** – internal feeling of knowing I will feel better about myself after exercising i.e. make it attractive.

3. The **response** – I put into action my five-minute rule (see page 173) so I start off by committing to just five minutes of exercise. My dumb-bells and exercise mat are not stored away so I am ready to go i.e. make it easy.

4. The **reward** – I feel energized for the day ahead and have a sense of accomplishment. I buy a coffee after the workout as a tangible reward i.e. make it satisfying.

And when trying to break bad habits, he advises that we invert the laws from positive to negative:

1. The **cue** – make it ~~obvious~~ invisible.

2. The **craving** – make it ~~attractive~~ unappealing.

3. The **response** – make it ~~easy~~ difficult.

4. The **reward** – make it ~~satisfying~~ unsatisfying.

Habit stacking

Trying to change habits or introduce new ones sounds simple on paper but it can be incredibly challenging to implement them. A simple and effective technique to incorporate new habits into your day is habit stacking. It basically means that you 'stack' the new behaviour on to a current behaviour to make you remember to do it, and so it just becomes part of your routine. It makes adopting a new habit into your routine much less overwhelming and it's more likely to become a lasting habit. Here are some examples:

You would like to drink more water, but you keep forgetting because your established habit is to drink tea throughout the day. Well, how about building a habit on top of the original habit? From now on, just before you fill the kettle, you drink a glass of water. After a while, you'll notice you do it as easily as filling the kettle.

If you have a habit of grabbing a sandwich every lunchtime, why not also grab an orange or an apple? Build extra nourishment into your daily routine.

If you always take a quick dip in the sea, build in a few stretches and yoga poses before you get in.

If you always go for a gentle stroll with your dog around the block, practise some mindful breathing at the same time.

You get the idea. This is how you habit stack. Eventually, with the new habit firmly in place, you can start to reduce and change the old ones, letting the new ones take over. Just be patient as it takes a lot longer for habits to form than you might think.

Lifestyle tweaks

'Don't judge each day by the harvest
you reap but by the seeds you plant'
— Robert Louis Stevenson

Let's work on what I call 'the tweaks'. The word 'change' can be so overwhelming. Often, we don't want or need to change our lifestyle, or our routines don't allow for a major overhaul due to family or work commitments. Don't put pressure on yourself to make huge changes — sometimes a little tweak is all that is necessary. Simply moving forward in the right direction towards your intended goal is more than enough.

A tweak could be what we discussed before — changing from a creamy latte to an Americano with warm milk, or walking the dog for an extra ten minutes. Don't start big, start so small you can't fail.

Once you get going, don't let it all go just because you don't turn up one time. Some days we are not operating at 100 per cent capacity, maybe not even 70 per cent. There are days we simply cannot turn up for ourselves, often because we are consumed with turning up for others. Don't scrap the walk because you 'don't have time'. Just do 10 per cent of what you would normally do. And consistently aim to show up in some way, in any way.

For me, I realized that snoozing the alarm can cause me to start off the day on the back foot. I end up rushing around because if I hit snooze once, it mightn't end there, so I don't snooze my alarm. Motivational speaker and author Mel

Robbins has a great tip called 'the five-second rule'. When you feel like you hesitate before doing something you know you should do, count back from five – and move. So, when that alarm goes off, I count back from five and then just get up. 5,4,3,2,1 and once you are up, you are up.

Another tweak I have made is to often try to park my car further away from where I need to go – a work meeting, shopping (except when grocery shopping), meeting a friend. This allows me to get extra steps into my day and up my general movement with little effort. The hardest part is remembering to do it!

My top-five tips for making lasting lifestyle tweaks:

- Don't base the tweaks you are making on what other people are doing. You are making the tweaks for YOU, not for anyone else.
- Look at the things that you want to make happen and shape habits around these.
- Think about what you would like your life to look like. Do these new habits work with this new version of your life?
- Go slow. Only change one habit at a time.
- Don't give up. If you forget to work on incorporating your new habit one day, try again. Consistently aim to show up in some way, in any way. It's not all or nothing.

The five-minute rule

On days when I'm not feeling it, I always say to myself, 'Just do five minutes, and if you don't want to continue, then don't.' It takes the pressure off. I always find that as soon as the five minutes are up, my attitude has changed to, 'Well, I've gone to the trouble of starting this now, I may as well keep going and finish it.'

This trick can be used for anything – studying for exams, a college assignment, doing a spring clean. What's needed is the motivation to start, then the process takes over. The five-minute rule will help you to start.

The key to all of this is applying it to your life. I can tell you what I do all day long and it won't make any difference to you if you don't incorporate it into your own lifestyle. I can tell you to lift weights regularly and eat breakfast, because I do those things and they work for me, but your interests, your genetics, your lifestyle will be different to mine. You need to create your own habits to fit your style of life.

14. The value of structure in making choices

'Through discipline comes freedom'
— Aristotle

The idea of having structure in your life is tied up with routine. Routines mean you know what to expect day to day, but building structure reflects your bigger life picture. Having structure in your life can improve productivity and reduce stress and anxiety. It creates a sense of stability and brings balance to your daily life.

You can build structure by committing to things, by having routines, by setting boundaries, prioritizing areas of your life and making good choices that work for you. It is an ever-flexible system, and you should sit down on a regular basis to evaluate what is working for you and what isn't.

At one point in time, I can safely say that my life lacked structure. And what happened? I burnt out. I think for a lot of people it's true to say that they feel other people are doing more or achieving more in their daily lives perhaps than they are. You know, the neighbour who has five kids, works full-time, has an Etsy side business selling homemade jewellery, still manages to get to the gym, is on the PTA and is training for a marathon, and seems to always be out and about meeting friends. And you can't help but think, 'Well, if they can, I should be able to too.'

But a lot comes into play in different people's lives, and you don't know what they are coping with – and what they are failing to cope with. Personality is a huge factor in how individual coping mechanisms work, and you can't compare your life to someone else's. Most importantly, you don't know the cost to someone of living how they do. Is striving to pack that much in causing them to miss out on the enjoyment part?

Until recent years, it was widely thought that people react to stress in the same way, and so if people looked okay, we decided that they *were* okay. Nowadays, thankfully, we know better. Burnout can manifest and show up in different ways depending on the individual. And not only that but there are different kinds of burnout, like that from overload, from neglect and from a lack of challenge.

I am someone who feels that I need to do things well every single time, and back in school I was incredibly hard on myself during exams, the same in college and the same in my sport and my work. I have always put huge amounts of pressure on myself.

When I left Cork and moved to Dublin, I did so knowing that I had taken a huge risk – I had left my job, my relationship, and retired from the Cork team – and so, with my sense of perfectionism, I couldn't bear to fail in my new venture. I wanted to prove to myself, and to everyone, that I had made the right choice. Underneath my enthusiasm was a strong feeling that I was about to be found out, which meant that I had a distinct worry around saying no, and so I said yes to everything.

Looking back, it was because I had left behind my old identity – Anna Geary, the Cork camogie player – and I was trying to figure out my new identity. The page was blank, I had to write the story. I also qualified in executive and performance coaching and was doing some corporate speaking, and I was afraid that if I said no to an offer, I would see all doors close.

Everything I was asked to do, I said yes to – every job, every charity event, every medal-giving ceremony, I said yes to all of them. And I found myself on the road, one day after the other, chasing my tail from Dublin to every county in Ireland because I didn't want to disappoint people. I didn't want people to think I thought I was better than their offer now that I had 'been on telly'.

I was bringing more and more into the box and never leaving anything out of it. I had no structure to my life; I had no downtime. I felt like I was in a pressure cooker, but with no valves open. The steam couldn't escape, and so it headed inward. I found myself getting upset easily and being uncharacteristically negative. I was irritable and found it hard to concentrate – my attention span was also affected. I felt demotivated when it came to training. I couldn't sleep or unwind. The quality of my sleep suffered because my mind wouldn't quieten down and I couldn't relax. I had burnt out.

Learning to set boundaries

Thankfully, one of the ways to pass as an executive coach is to be coached yourself, and in those sessions I learned a little bit about coping and took on a skillset I didn't have before. I learned to set boundaries. I told myself I couldn't take on every job, and I prioritized my downtime as a necessity for health. I started to say no to things I didn't want to do, so that I could leave the way open for the things that moved me closer to my goals and passions.

Reducing stress and avoiding burnout isn't easy, especially when often we feel we have to keep going. Stress can overwhelm our system and makes everything harder and more challenging; the very impact of the stress response makes the problem feel more intense and makes coping with it far more difficult. When our mind is racing and our heart rate is up, sitting calmly and figuring anything out is not easy.

So, what do we do? Sometimes we make a drastic change, completely overhaul our eating habits, or start an intense exercise programme with great intentions. We swear we will make that leap (*I'll start Monday!*), sometimes we open up the job-hunting pages online, or randomly start digging up the garden for the pond we always said we would do if we had the time, and never make any changes at all. I have fallen into this trap myself. The answer is to build structure and routine into your life, prioritizing what's important, staying committed to your goals and making good choices that work for you.

Implementing structure in your life

There are parts of everyone's life that work, and parts of our lives that don't work. We need to be able to assess which areas aren't working and would benefit from a change.

Let's take the analogy of a cutlery drawer for a moment and use it to describe the different components of health (physical exercise, hydration, sleep, mental well-being, rest and down-time). Think about the cutlery drawer in your kitchen. You have tablespoons, forks, knives, teaspoons, sharp knives, all there to serve different purposes. You can't eat soup or cereal with a knife, so having loads of knives isn't much good if you don't have any spoons.

The same can be said for your health. If you exercise five days a week, while that is great, it isn't much good to your overall health if you only get five hours of sleep a night, or if you neglect drinking water. It's about putting a bit of structure on things and reflecting on what's working and what's not working. Drill down into what you find. Why are you exercising so much and sleeping so little? Can you give up an early-morning spin class for an extra hour's sleep perhaps?

Take a page in your journal and put a line down the middle. On one side write down the areas in life that work, and on the other, those that are not working. Do this once a month if possible. I've written a few examples of what you might include.

What's working	What's not working
· Weekly meet-up with the girls · Getting up an hour earlier to walk the dog in the morning · Prepping a salad to bring to work each day	· No time to see my parents · Having to use the car too much · Sleep patterns all over the place

By exploring what is currently working for you and what's not, you can identify where you need to make necessary improvements or tweaks. It might give you a better sense of control and help reduce any stress and anxiety you may have if you're currently not giving yourself enough time to do something important – like choosing to binge on *Real Housewives* rather than meeting with a friend for a walk in the evening. See if you can swap out the negative with the positive. This all leads on to the concept of prioritizing.

Why we need to prioritize

'The key is not to prioritize what's on your schedule, but to schedule your priorities'
– Stephen R. Covey

I think it's safe to say that most of us live busy lives of distraction. Our timetables feel packed and yet we are spending more time on social media than ever. We seem to spend hours in the car and we get stuck in this rolling ball of commute, desk, commute, couch and eventually bed. Repeat. And while we know this isn't good for us, we don't prioritize investing in our future selves right now.

We need to prioritize certain things and we need to make time work for us, rather than against us. If we don't prioritize, then everything becomes urgent. We suffer from burnout, we can't work out how to alleviate the stress, and it takes a toll on our mental, physical and emotional health.

Role priority list

Rather than focusing on the never-ending 'To Do' list, why not try making a role priority list? Think about all the roles you play in your life – parent, partner, brother, sister, friend, student, grandchild, neighbour, charity worker, teammate, boss, colleague . . . the list goes on. Most of us play many different roles and we often have to wear multiple, interchangeable hats. First, take a moment to congratulate yourself because you fulfil a lot of different roles in your life. Sometimes some can take priority over others. How do you decide what takes preference? Try this:

At weekends, I always take a few minutes to think about the roles I may need to fulfil in the coming week. What is coming up for me? A family occasion, so I am in daughter or mum mode? An exam, so I am in student mode? A work deadline, so I am in work mode? Then I list the roles in order of importance for the week ahead.

And sometimes you need to make a priority decision

when something unexpected comes up. Years ago, when I was first dating my now husband, I was also studying for an important exam in which I wanted to do well. In the middle of one of my final study sessions, I received a phone call from Kev's teammate telling me that Kev had sustained an injury during a match and had to go to hospital for an X-ray.

Typically, something like this would be a dilemma as you'd have to stop and deliberate what to do, thus wasting time and valuable energy. But this is where the role priority list came into play. We must have been getting on particularly well that week because I had my role of girlfriend ranked higher than student in my list of priorities at the time! Going to the hospital took precedence over the studying. By identifying the roles, you know what comes first in your day or week and it makes subsequent decisions easier.

Identifying what makes you happy

Take your journal and, using the prompts, finish the sentences below. Don't think too long or hard about this, the answer is usually the first that springs to mind.

- I feel great about life when . . .
- On my perfect day off I would . . .
- The five things I wish I had more time for are . . .

Making better choices

'May your choices reflect your hopes not your fears'
— Nelson Mandela

Think about the choices you've made in your daily life that you know weren't the right ones for you. What ways do you use time, what do you eat, what do you do, that you know is not bringing you fulfilment and a sense of satisfaction? Maybe you'll think of the takeaway you had last night. Maybe you regret getting it and wish you'd cooked something healthy from scratch instead. Does it happen more often than not? You've come in after a long day, you're tired, and instead of going to the bother of cooking, you choose the easy option, and then you lie in bed wishing you had just made an omelette instead. This is the result of a lack of structure.

When you structure your life, even in a gentle way, you are less likely to regret your decisions. You have thought through your choices for that day and aligned them with the values and the life that you want.

When it comes to making better choices, we just need to check in to make sure they are serving us. Ask yourself 'Will this nourish me today?' It's such a simple question. Will it nourish my body? Will it nourish my mind? Will it nourish my soul?

Sometimes when you are faced with a decision and you ask that question, you will end up deciding against the takeaway and making something healthier from your already-stocked fridge instead. Sometimes you won't. Sometimes you will decide to cancel the run and jump on to the couch to indulge in some well-deserved R&R. Sometimes you won't. But don't make the easy option your default choice. Make considered, conscious decisions.

Do more, do less, do differently – an exercise to help you reflect

Reflection is a good way to challenge your thinking and actions. It lets you take stock of what you are actually doing. Sometimes what we think, and then do, doesn't match up. Here is an exercise that can be done as a short wind-down, preparing for the next day or for the next week. Divide a page into three columns: *Do more/Do less/Do differently.*

- **What do you want to do more of?** It could be to get more exercise or more sleep or get out into nature.
- **What do you want to do less of?** Say, scrolling social media at night or grazing instead of eating proper balanced meals.
- And of the things you currently do, **what do you want to do differently?** You might be staying in touch with loved ones, but maybe the conversation is always negative or bitchy – are you constantly giving out about a particular person? Do you want to change the chat to a different tone? Or maybe you are showing up to exercise classes, but you are

always rushing in last minute, a bit frantic, perhaps missing some of the warm-up as a result (I'm nodding in agreement for this one!).

You can pick as many things as you like under each heading but be realistic as it's about implementing changes.

Alongside each of your findings above, write down one action step you can take to help. For example, scrolling social media at night – *put a timer on my phone to lock certain apps after a particular time.* Being on time for gym classes – *prepare gear in advance so I'm not searching for it, and leave five minutes earlier than usual.* It's just about taking a different approach.

Make better choices with your time

Sit down and work out how much of your day is taken up by sleep, work, commute, cleaning, family obligations, etc. Try to figure out the actual way you're spending your time. I guarantee you that you will find huge pockets of time left over. Yet so many of us tell ourselves 'I don't have time' when it comes to looking after our health, nurturing our relationships, practising self-care or whatever it is you tell yourself you don't have time for.

There will be at least two or three hours that can be classed as free time. What are you currently doing with it? Binge-watching a series on TV? Aimlessly scrolling on social media?

Now think – what would you like to be doing with that

time? Two spare hours every day is fourteen hours a week to spend with your kids, your parents, your friends . . . to exercise, to take up a hobby, to plan new goals and make new decisions. Stop telling yourself you don't have time. And remember, if you have time to scroll, then you have time to stroll.

If you do one thing every morning, do this!

We see so much online about morning routines, but if you make one addition to your morning, let this be it. Replace the use of your phone in the first fifteen minutes of your day with something else. Anything else. Reading, journalling, stretching, meditation, making a cup of coffee. Or even just allowing yourself the space to wake up and ease yourself into the day.

Many of us use our phones as an alarm clock. Picture the scene. Your alarm beeps and you turn it off. The phone is in your hand, whether it's a conscious decision or not, while you are in the process of waking up. With one eye blearily open and your head still on the pillow, you swipe across and open your phone.

Suddenly, you are reading the news, reading texts and emails, or scrolling social media. You are looking at everything people are doing, or what people need from you. Someone has posted a picture of a sunrise hike or has already showered after their morning run. Maybe you are watching a story about someone having the kids' lunches cut into star shapes, or you read an email from a person who is already at work. The voice in your head is shouting, 'Why aren't you doing that? You aren't even up yet!'

Before you've even sat up in the bed and put your two feet on the ground, you are dictating how your day is going to start – which is in a reactive state. Your levels of cortisol (stress hormone) begin to rise, and you can start to get a sickening feeling growing in your stomach that you are somehow already behind, chasing the day.

Do yourself a favour: ditch the phone. Leave it outside your bedroom door or at least on the other side of the room out of reach. But what about the alarm clock, I hear you say? Once upon a time, there were these things that existed called digital alarm clocks that you put on your bedside table. You can still get them. It will be the best €10 you will spend on your health. Give yourself the gift of spending those few minutes focusing on yourself, not focusing on what anyone else is doing.

The power of no

'Saying "yes" to one thing means saying "no" to another. That's why decisions can be hard sometimes'
– Sean Covey

As you can probably tell from my story of burnout, I have experienced first-hand the fear of saying no. Saying no to people is one of the more difficult things to do, so we avoid it and end up rushing around trying to fit everything in and please everyone. Our life has no structure, chaos abounds, and we become stressed and even anxious. Sound familiar?

It is important to understand that when you say yes to something or someone, you are saying no to something else. Maybe it's your goals, your health, your downtime. Think of the last time you said yes to something you really didn't want to do, but you didn't want to let someone down. By saying yes, what did you say no to? Was it time with your kids, the hot bath you'd been dreaming of for days, or was it no to exercise because you didn't have the time?

What are you willing to tolerate in your life? Disappointing others on occasion, so that you can prioritize your own life? Are you always making decisions based on the fear of letting someone else down? Yes, there are some things we need to do, but saying no is sometimes what we need to do. We need to do it for ourselves, and we need to do it to set an example to others.

How to say no

It's still a work in progress for me, but one tip I have learned is that if you have to say no, do not put it off. Don't tell people you'll let them know, or to check back in a few days, unless you have to genuinely think about it. Don't mislead them or procrastinate about giving them an answer. All it does is make it harder for you to say no eventually.

When saying no, be honest and direct. Don't leave room for any ambiguity.

Now, this is important – never say yes if you know you are going to renege on it later. That is far worse than saying no to begin with.

Another thing I have learned when it comes to saying no is that it's not what you say, it's how you say it. While you can be direct, the language you use doesn't have to be needlessly harsh or rude. Don't overexplain yourself either – if you have to say no then you have to say no.

Taking back the option of saying no can be quite empowering. It enables you to make a choice on how to structure your day, your week, your life, in a way that best suits you.

Fight, flight or freeze response

Our (autonomic) nervous system is vital to achieving balance when it comes to our well-being. It is comprised of two parts: the sympathetic and the parasympathetic nervous systems, which have opposite roles. Our sympathetic nervous system carries signals that put our bodies' systems on high alert and activates our fight, flight or freeze response during potential danger. In contrast, our parasympathetic nervous system's job is to carry signals that relax and restore our bodies to a sense of calm, or back into 'rest and digest' mode.

When your fight, flight or freeze response is activated, cortisol and adrenaline are both released in your body as your brain goes into protective mode. Your body responds accordingly. Your heart rate can increase. It can cause sweaty palms or your pupils to dilate, and the hairs on your body to stand up. Your breathing quickens and often becomes shallower too. Interestingly, it also slows body processes that are less important in emergencies, such as digestion, which is why you can feel bloated when you're stressed.

All of this can create the illusion of being under threat. And this in turn elicits the same response early humans would have experienced when they were being charged at by a wild animal.

Here's the thing we must understand: our brain cannot distinguish between different types of danger – it doesn't know what caused the perceived threat, it just knows the body's signals. Centuries ago, it might have been trying to hide from a predatory animal, but in today's world it could be a nasty comment on social media, or a confrontational email from a colleague. But the chemical response in the body is the same whenever our fight, flight or freeze mode is activated.

We are not designed to stay in this state for long periods of time but because a lot of us are living in a perpetual state of stress, we may be in this fight, flight or freeze mode more than we should. This can lead to chronic stress and burnout.

If you are feeling stressed or burnt out, I suggest trying the exercises below to help restore some sense of calm.

Now, we are not trying to eliminate all pressure and stress from our lives. Aside from the fact that it would be almost impossible to do so, we must remember that a certain amount of pressure, and even stress, is necessary for us in life. Usually, the concept of pressure can carry negative connotations and people are speaking negatively when they say 'I'm under pressure'. However, pressure can be an ally and is sometimes even a motivating factor. It can help us to push ourselves to achieve our goals and rise to the occasion in certain circumstances. It allows us to meet deadlines, sit exams and engage in public speaking. The trick is to keep the pressure in check so that it doesn't become excessive, and to have coping mechanisms in place for when the pressure and in turn the stress get too much.

Exercises for stress reduction

Well-being is ultimately about 'being well' in your mind and your body. How often do you check in with yourself and ask: *How do I feel? What are my energy levels like today?*

Do it right now. Take a moment. Rate your current energy levels between 1 and 10. Be honest with yourself but refrain from feeling any guilt or judgement. Once you have decided on the number (don't think about it for too long), then ask yourself a valuable question: *What can I do today to improve this number by just 1?*

So, to take it from a 1 to a 2, or a 5 to a 6, depending on where you are on the scale, it could be something like:

- Ringing someone for a catch-up
- Listening to your favourite song and dancing around the kitchen
- Asking a friend for help
- Getting out for a walk
- Making your favourite dinner

Whatever it is, do it! You know it will make you feel better. Some other simple things to do, if you don't have much time to increase your energy and lower your stress, are the two following exercises.

Sixty-second mindful minute

This is a functional exercise, focusing on our breath – it is not meditation. Personally, I find it hard to meditate, but this exercise is more about the biomechanics of breathing.

When we are stressed, our breathing quickens, we sigh more, breathing becomes shallower – and we fall into the trap of chest breathing, instead of breathing from our bellies.

Now, notice how you are sitting. Make sure your feet are fully flat on the floor. Take your shoes off if you want to. Think about your posture – shoulders back and down. Open up your airway. Place one palm on your chest and one palm on your belly. When you inhale through your nose, notice if your belly is filling up with air or is just your chest rising? Focus on trying to fill your belly with air, like a balloon. Slowly inhale for four seconds, hold for two seconds, slowly and deeply exhale for four seconds. Do this six times – that's sixty seconds.

Slowing down your breathing actively sends a signal to your brain that everything is okay. You are not in danger. This breathing technique can help you to retreat into 'rest and digest' mode.

Shake it out

This exercise helps with nervous system regulation.

Get up and move around. Start by tightening and releasing your fists. Then consciously try to tighten and shake out different muscles and parts of your body, including your arms and legs, and simply shake. This shaking movement is scientifically proven to release built-up tension in our bodies.

Whether it's a feeling of anger, irritation, anxiety or being overwhelmed with life, release it.

Shaking activates the parasympathetic nervous system and sends signals to the brain to calm, relax and let go.

Rest and recharge

We don't tend to place the same emphasis on rest and recovery as we do on the 'go, go, go' mentality. We are human beings, but it often feels like we are human *doings*. If you have a phone you will know you have to charge it up every night or the battery will be flat the next day when you need it. Your phone has so many crucial functions which are necessary for your life to run efficiently each day – your wallet, contact numbers, emails, etc.

But what about your body and mind? Do they both not perform essential functions daily? If we don't recharge them, they too will go flat, and yet often recharging our phone seems more important. What if we paid the same attention to the battery life of our bodies and minds? Right now, how does your body battery feel? Do you need a quick charge? Try the exercises above for starters.

193

15. Tactics board for consistency

'When you're so consistent, people have to stand up
and take notice. I don't think people recognize or
praise consistency enough'
— Katie Taylor

One of the most important values you can have in life is
consistency. It enables you to show up for yourself and for
other people. It allows you to be the best version of you. In
being consistent, you have made a commitment to the goals
you have set for yourself, allowing you to feel purposeful in
your day-to-day life. By implementing a structure to your
life – encompassing a solid routine and positive habits – it
will make it easier for you to consistently strive to achieve
your goals. Surround yourself with a good support system,
become more conscious in your decision-making and learn
to set boundaries for yourself. These factors will all help you
live a more fulfilled and active life.

Anna's take-home points

- Make a solid commitment to achieving your goals by writing an action plan and putting a strong support system in place. Banish negative self-talk. You can do it!
- Maximize your routine so that you can focus on what you really want to achieve.
- Small tweaks to habits can have a profound effect on your life. Find out what you want to change, and make it happen.
- Is your life structured in a way that works for you? If not, change it up. Set boundaries, make conscious choices, know what your priorities are.
- Learn how to say no.

Read

Atomic Habits – James Clear
The High 5 Habit – Mel Robbins
Mind Full – Dermot Whelan
Just One Thing – Dr Michael Mosley
The Burnout Solution – Siobhán Murray
Legacy – James Kerr
Commit! – Enda McNulty

Listen

Real Health With Karl Henry podcast
The Food Medic podcast – Dr Hazel Wallace
The Good Glow podcast – Georgie Crawford

Watch

The Pursuit of Happyness
Cast Away
The Devil Wears Prada
Rush
Formula 1: Drive to Survive

Notes

Consistency – my personal tactics board

....

....

....

....

....

....

....

....

....

....

....

PART FOUR

Game Plan for Challenge

16. What makes us stronger

'You never know how strong you are,
until being strong is your only choice'

– Bob Marley

Wouldn't it be great if we could glide gracefully through life with no obstacles to hinder our path? Sadly, nothing is ever perfect, and challenges are part and parcel of our daily lives. It is *how* we cope with the hurdles in life that makes us stronger. I firmly believe that challenges in our life can be used to our advantage. Each one presents an opportunity for personal growth and self-improvement. Challenges can help you develop strength and resilience, and they can teach you how to fail and how to pick yourself up again.

When you achieve what you set out to do, despite the setbacks, the missteps and the unforeseen circumstances, the sense of accomplishment that you will experience will be incredible. Challenges make the prize all the sweeter – even though it might not seem like it at the time! For me, I think there are two types of challenges: you can be challenged and you can set yourself a challenge. One is outside of your control; one is more controllable. However, both will take you out of your comfort zone.

When I found out my dad was terminally ill in 2022, it shook me to my core. I remember exactly where I was and exactly what I was doing at the time my phone rang with the news. If you have ever had to experience this, you will be able to relate. A random Tuesday in February, a significant day in my life for ever. That same week I was presenting *Supercharged*, a live health and well-being radio show on RTÉ Radio 1, and the main discussion topic was one I had fought hard for in our production meeting a few weeks previously. A necessary, uncomfortable, universal subject – grief and bereavement.

As I prepared in the days leading up to the show, the content in my briefs took on a whole new meaning. The questions became more pertinent than ever. Only a select few people knew that my dad was ill. There was a multitude of obvious reasons not to cover the topic at a time when I had received such devastating news, but for me it somehow felt more important than ever to go ahead with it.

All the feelings and thoughts experienced in the build-up to the show had to be compartmentalized. I had to do my job as a broadcaster and facilitate the conversations with the experts on the show as best I could. I had a duty to hold it together, to overcome the challenge of allowing my emotions to creep in, to maximize the value of the content and advice for the audience. It was a remarkably powerful show, albeit probably the greatest challenge I have faced in my professional career. I was incredibly proud to present it.

17. Challenge yourself

'Challenge yourself.
It's the only path which leads to growth'
— Morgan Freeman

Growth mindset versus fixed mindset

When I work with corporate groups, one of the things that comes up a lot for people looking to progress in their careers is the idea of a growth mindset versus a fixed mindset. This concept is the work of Carol Dweck in her renowned book *Mindset: The New Psychology of Success*, and I will give you a brief snapshot of what it means in terms of the challenges we face, and how you might be able to apply it to your life.

Someone with a fixed mindset tends to believe that their intelligence and talents are fixed – they know what they know, and they have nothing more to learn. As a result, they neglect the impact that effort, further learning and perseverance can have in their life. They tend to avoid challenges and prefer staying in their comfort zone. They are also more likely to engage in negative self-talk, which we know from earlier chapters is key to hindering self-growth.

205

On the other hand, a person who has a growth mindset believes that their intelligence and talents can be developed over time. They embrace learning opportunities and know the benefits of hard work, they take on new challenges and are more likely to engage in constructive self-talk.

The key differences between those with growth versus fixed mindsets:

	Fixed	Growth
Challenges	Avoid	Embrace
Obstacles	Give up easily	Persist
Effort	Pointless	Imperative
Criticism	Ignore	Take on board and learn
Success	Threatened by others' success	Inspired by and find lessons in others' success
Result	Achieve less than their full potential	High level of achievement

Maybe by simply looking at these comparisons, we can start to identify what sort of mindset we have. The trap we can fall into is to wrongly assume that because we identify with one aspect of a growth mindset, we *have* a growth mindset. But then, when you drill into it, other aspects like 'take on board criticism' or 'embrace stepping out of your comfort zone' may not be as applicable.

206

No matter where you are when it comes to mindset, look for the evidence. Challenge your thinking. The question is: *How do we transform our fixed mindset into a growth mindset?*

One way to do this is to identify triggers from our past. We are all products of our childhoods, and our experiences help shape us to become the people we are now. Our minds have an enormous capacity to hold on to memories. Try to reflect on past influences and they may shed some light on limiting beliefs or a self-defeating outlook. Maybe you had a bad experience in school, and you were told that you couldn't achieve something? Maybe you were bullied at one point, and you now shy away from anything that could draw attention to you? Maybe you were criticized for your weight, and it made you feel worthless? All these things could close your mind off to embracing challenges and moving forward.

Instead, turn these triggers into an opportunity for growth by using the following strategies:

- **Reframe past experiences** – try to think of a benefit or a positive in that experience that you had not previously considered.
- **Recognize your own potential for growth and learning** – despite any adversity you may have experienced in the past.
- **Adopt a more proactive approach to overcoming challenges** – maybe break down the challenge into smaller steps and make an action plan.

If you start understanding yourself a little bit more through some self-reflection, you might be able to tackle challenges with more self-belief. It's not easy, but why not try?

When I finished college, I applied for a graduate training programme with a prominent company. I was excited about it – I remember thinking, *This could be it, my future workplace.* The interview was a whole-day affair. We had to deliver a presentation, do a formal interview and take part in team-building exercises with the other candidates. I did all the research and put so much work into the presentation.

The day was exhausting. I knew I was ready and prepared and also that I was a good team player, so I went in with a positive attitude. After the interview day, I was feeling quietly confident. I felt it had gone well. You can imagine my dismay when I received a rejection letter a couple of weeks later. It really knocked me.

The thing was, what I had believed – that I had performed well – and what the company wanted, weren't the same. I couldn't see that at the time. I thought that suitability was the same as doing well. But, of course, that's not the truth. A lot of things come into play when companies are choosing employees, but the rejection I felt was huge. The reason I was so knocked back was that I had tied my self-worth to the job, and getting the job was validation that I was good enough.

The sense of rejection, of not being good enough, was a feeling and experience that I had to reframe to give myself the courage to move forward and go for the next job. I had to believe that going through the process was a learning

208

experience, and I took it with me when I moved onwards. What I learned from this experience and what I always try to remember is: *Whether something works out or not, it doesn't detract from who you are as a person.* Now repeat that five times.

The practical application of a growth mindset

'Keep challenging yourself to think better,
do better, and be better'
– Robin Sharma

So, now we're working on a growth mindset, how do we utilize that in everyday life? What can we learn, what challenges can we undertake, that will push us towards our goals, whether personal or professional? And how do we do this?

I'm going to talk about this specifically in relation to fitness and exercise, but you can just as easily apply these concepts to other parts of your life.

These days, it is easy to live a sedentary life – we can work from home, we have every streaming service available for our entertainment needs, and oftentimes social media replaces real interaction. So, unlike our ancestors, who moved all day out of necessity, we need to build exercise into our routines more. We need to prioritize it. And this in itself is a challenge in our busy lives. I'm telling you now, you won't regret it – movement, whether basic exercise or sport, is so beneficial, mentally, physically and emotionally.

I'll start on Monday

We always do this – procrastinate. It's human nature. We want to implement the change, but for some reason we feel the need to schedule it for a future date. Maybe it's next Monday, maybe it's the New Year (*New Year, New You* anyone?); either way, we tend to put lifestyle changes off indefinitely. But remember what I was telling you about taking baby steps? It's important to just get going, and to stack new habits: take the stairs now, not on Monday, walk to work today, not next month. Start today, immediately.

In terms of health and fitness, the New Year is a time when we all make resolutions. And, of course, it is a time when a lot of us feel like failures, our resolutions fading away into the reality of the habits and lifestyle we already have. We said this year would be the year, this year would be different, this year we would have no excuses . . . but then we find ourselves struggling, we launch in hard and give up quickly, the brand-new bike gathering dust in the shed and the running gear shoved to the back of the wardrobe. Why does this happen?

Generally, the goal we set is too big – *I'll go cycling every day for an hour* – without considering if that's viable, or too vague – *I'll get fit* – but with no concrete plan. And so we procrastinate, and the vicious circle continues – we're too lazy, too unfit, we've failed again, adopting a 'can't change, won't change' mentality.

We need to reframe exercise in our head, retrain our brain to think that activity and movement will nourish our body, our heart, our lungs. It will nourish our muscles, strengthening and toning them, and it will nourish our souls, making us feel great about ourselves simply by taking part. We are led to believe that we need to be out of breath, maxing out or sweating buckets to be exercising, and sometimes we will do that, but gentle exercise, simply moving your body in whatever way works for you, is just as important too.

It can be a real challenge to retrain how we feel about exercise, but it is worth it. Exercise because you respect your body, not because you want to punish it.

How not to procrastinate:

- **Do something you enjoy** – whether that's going for a walk with a friend, going along to a yoga class, taking up tennis or going out for a run. If you enjoy it, you're more likely to do it. And the more you do it, the better you'll feel.
- **Make a solid date** – whether that's signing up for a class you must commit to, or scheduling it into your daily routine, make sure it's something that is difficult to cancel.
- **Make it social** – if you can do exercise with other people, all the better. Remember, they will hold you accountable if you don't show up! But they will also praise you when you do, or when you hit your goal.
- **Have an achievable, specific goal** – as we explored previously, if your fitness goal is too big, or vague, it's less likely that you will keep at it. Have an achievable goal and you're much more likely to commit to it.

Step outside your comfort zone

'All growth starts at the end of your comfort zone'
– Tony Robbins

They say the comfort zone is the place where we perform something to a steady level, without a sense of risk. It's those times when you are running but not pushing it, eating the food you know you like but might not be the best for you, staying at the job that pays okay and doesn't ask too much of you.

Some comfort zones are good things, they give us a sense of security and stability. But sometimes we get stuck in them and can't figure a way out, leaving us feeling burnt out and demotivated. Our brain loves the comfort zone, because, as we well know, it loves familiar things and operating on autopilot, but if we stay in that zone for too long, we lose any chance of self-growth. We need challenges to push us for our own good – whether it's physical or mental.

If you push past the comfort zone, through the fear zone, you will step into the growth zone, where you become someone seeking out the best for yourself and where you can live out your dreams. Intentionally leaving the comfort zone is tied in with developing a growth mindset – the two go hand in hand. By challenging yourself, you open yourself up to new opportunities, new ways to live and to be.

This diagram* is useful to help you visualize the different stages of leaving the comfort zone and moving into a growth zone.

Moving from your comfort to your growth zone

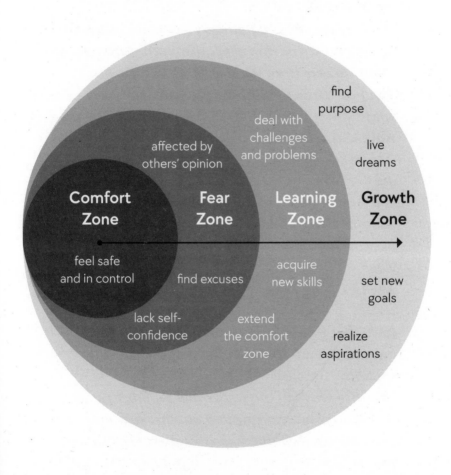

* Adapted from PositivePsychology.com Toolkit – 'Leaving the Comfort Zone'

The zones explained:

- **The Comfort Zone** – this is where you like to be (you think). It's secure, you feel in control because everything is familiar, and no real demands are made of you.
  You have the same routine every day which allows for no time to exercise. You notice that you're getting out of breath quicker when you're walking up the stairs.

- **The Fear Zone** – this is the scary second stage where you will start to feel anxious and fearful. You make excuses, you procrastinate, and you will likely start facing challenges that you did not have in the comfort zone.
  You join the gym, but you are worried. What if everyone is really fit and looks better than you? Do you have the right gear? What if you can't keep up in the class?

- **The Learning Zone** – you've pushed through the fear. Well done! You're on your way! You begin to learn about the new venture you have embarked on, and you are acquiring the skillset needed to overcome the challenge.
  You go to the gym. You realize that the other people in your class are simply trying their best, like you, and just go to improve their fitness and clear their head for an hour.

- **The Growth Zone** – you learn to set new goals, and have confidence to try to achieve them, regardless of how well you do. You have new skills; you know your strengths and you use them to achieve the best outcome for you.

The gym becomes somewhere that you regularly and willingly attend. You see an improvement in your fitness levels, and you can now lift heavier weights in your classes.

Getting out of your comfort zone

Reframing uncomfortable experiences

Think back to times in your life when you have had to step out of your comfort zone, whether you wanted to or not. Going to college? Moving away from home? Going out on a first date? New job? Now ask yourself:

How did you feel?
What happened?
How did you cope?
Can you think of any lessons to take from it?

If you're stranded in your comfort zone, unsure of how to take the first steps towards leading a more fulfilled life in the growth zone, you might find the following suggestions helpful:

- **Change your routine** – we looked at the benefits of changing your routine in chapter 13, and I just wanted to reiterate how important it is to switch things up to break yourself out of a comfortable, safe routine. They can be small changes. Turn off your phone by a certain time. Have dinner at the table instead of in front of the TV. Do five minutes of yoga in the morning instead of scrolling through news feeds. Small changes can be the most meaningful.

- **Try new recipes** – bring home new vegetables to cook and fruits to try. Pre-prepare meals and batch cook when you can.

- **Incorporate exercise into your life** – when it comes to stepping outside your comfort zone, thinking about it is often worse than doing. Don't be afraid to try out new exercises. You might discover your new favourite pastime. Look how many people have taken up sea swimming in the past few years, simply because they gave it a go and realized how much they enjoyed it. Get some friends involved and make it social.

- **Be honest with yourself** – this can be a huge challenge and is likely to take you out of your comfort zone. Writing your honest thoughts and feelings down in a journal can lead you on the road to personal growth.

The uncomfortable list

Make an 'uncomfortable' list. Write down ten things that make you feel uncomfortable and pick a new one to try out every week. Pick things from all different aspects of your life. For example . . .

Cycling instead of getting the bus
Trying kefir yoghurt instead of normal yoghurt
Volunteering to do a presentation at work
Organizing a neighbours' night out

Tell a friend about the list so they can hold you accountable to make sure you work through it.

What finding fault says about you

Sometimes when we are feeling vulnerable, feeling lost, unsure, or wishing things could be different, we find it hard – triggering, even – to see other people doing well. We may find ourselves remarking on others, finding fault or, dare I say it, hoping something goes wrong.

Since we can all scrutinize and put others down, is it any wonder that we can turn on ourselves and rip ourselves apart? No wonder we focus on our bodies and what we think is wrong with them. No wonder we are worried about putting ourselves out there outside of our comfort zone – even though deep down we really want to – because we know what we might say about someone else in the same position or because we are afraid to try, afraid to fail.

It is normal to feel like this, but you do need to become aware of this behaviour if you find yourself slipping into it. We cannot feel contentment internally if we are tearing people apart externally. It also inhibits us from trying new things. Remember, it rarely has anything to do with the person you are commenting on, it's more a projection of your own insecurities about where you are in your life, how you feel about yourself and your own progress. If you can become aware of something, you can control it; if you can control it, you can work towards changing it. It all starts with awareness.

On the pitch or on the sidelines?

In a sporting context, we are all capable of being the person watching on from the sidelines, commenting on the players on the pitch. Stating how things *should* be done, or how you would have played better. The person who talks about certain players not deserving their place on the team. The person who tears into managers for their decisions, insults the referee for wrong calls and criticizes the players for making mistakes. We all know someone like this. Begrudging nitpickers, as I like to call them.

And do you know what? These people will never be on the pitch. They never risk playing *in* the game. They remain where they are because it is safe, on the sidelines and in the stands. In their comfort zone. From a place of passive observation, they can feel better by thinking that they know what others should and shouldn't be doing. They can't fail that way. They won't get actively involved and risk failing at it, so they never try.

The same is true for life. It is easy to sit it out, to stay on the sidelines and criticize those who are having a go. We only get one shot, and my hope for you is that with this game plan you will no longer be simply a spectator in your own life and instead you will start to play the game.

Make the decision today: *Do you want to be the person on the pitch or the person on the sidelines?* Because you can become the player – the one doing it, getting stuck in, making mistakes, giving it a go, *trying*! We don't grow by achieving new things. We grow by *trying* new things. Courage is born from the act of trying, not achieving.

I have this famous quote from Theodore Roosevelt's 'Man in the Arena' speech framed and hanging up in my hallway at home:

> It is not the critic who counts . . . The credit belongs
> to the man who is actually in the arena, whose face
> is marred by dust and sweat and blood; who strives
> valiantly; who errs, who comes short again and
> again, because there is no effort without error and
> shortcoming.

This is a reminder to me that I'd rather be on the pitch,

in the game, trying and making the mistakes, than merely commenting on it as it passes me by.

When *Ireland's Fittest Family* is airing, I often see comments criticizing the efforts and the choices made by the families. Everyone's an expert on the couch. 'Oh, we could do that better,' or 'Why are they even on the show?' Every year, the families participating admit in their post-event chats that the challenges look so much easier when they are watching them on TV. The families that watch the show, and then decide to put themselves to the test – they're my kind of people. To put yourself out there, despite the fear. There is no courage in commenting.

Above all, remember: *Dimming someone else's light doesn't make yours shine brighter.*

Just do it

Think about something that you would like to try but are currently sitting on the sidelines instead. Maybe it's setting up a social media page for your business, going back to college, trying a new style of dressing. What is holding you back? You might see someone else doing something you reckon you would be good at, so instead of finding fault, go do it too.

Just say yes

'Start with a "Yes" and see where that takes you'
— Tina Fey

Saying yes to opportunities and challenges all ties in with developing your growth mindset and leaving your comfort zone. Saying yes can be truly transformative and can open your life up in different directions.

I remember when I was first asked to be a coach on *Ireland's Fittest Family* in 2015, I didn't know what to think. I had very limited experience in a coaching role apart from taking the odd training session with underage camogie teams. My mind flooded with all the reasons I shouldn't do it. Would I be shown up by the other coaches? What if I didn't get my strategies right? What if my coaching style didn't work on the show? How would I come across on TV in the heat of battle?

I could have easily said no, but I was curious. It was my first opportunity to get involved in a TV show, so I ignored the voice in my head and gave myself the nudge to go for it. Eight seasons and three wins later and I still adore the show. I genuinely get so invested in the families and I have learned so much about myself in the process. To think I almost missed that opportunity. And if I had said no, I would have always wondered *What if. . .?*

In chapter 14, and later in chapter 22, I talk about how saying no in certain situations can help you maintain boundaries, learn to prioritize and put yourself and your needs first. Saying yes in this context means still putting yourself first, but in a positive way. It is not about people-pleasing. It is about considering challenges that align with your goals and can present you with growth opportunities. The idea of saying yes may fill you with fear, and I will be addressing this in more detail in the next chapter. But you must reframe your mindset. This quick visualization might help:

Imagine what will happen if you say yes.

Then imagine what will happen if you say no.

How do you feel when you think about what might happen if you say yes? Is the fear overtaken by stirring feelings of excitement? If so, reframe it in your mind. You are not scared, you are excited!

In the next month, do something that makes you nervous, something you are not confident about. Maybe it's going for a night away on your own. Maybe it's booking into a new class without your friend by your side. Maybe it's applying for a work promotion. Try it. What have you got to lose?

Saying yes requires a certain level of work, commitment and determination. But think where it might take you.

And what happens if you say no? You're stuck where you were and will never know what you could have achieved.

365 days of yes

Saying yes is often harder to do than we realize, but it can be so rewarding. Set yourself the challenge of saying yes to something every day for a year. It doesn't have to be a yes to something big, it's more about saying yes to something that you might otherwise say no to.

For example, saying yes to picking up a new vegetable on your food shop and cooking it for dinner. Saying yes to starting a different genre of book. Saying yes to going on a date or trying out a new class. There are endless options and you just need to choose one thing every day.

Think about all the things you will have said yes to in a year's time. You may open new doors and have new experiences because of a simple daily yes. You might uncover a new favourite pastime or meet the love of your life while on a date.

Your first yes? Say *yes* to this challenge!

The jealousy compass

Mel Robbins is one of my favourite authors and motivational speakers. I love her no-nonsense attitude and she has certainly helped me to challenge my own thoughts and belief systems. In particular, she has an interesting way of looking at jealousy and, because of her, I have *tried* to change the way I interpret jealousy.

We have been conditioned to think about jealousy as a negative thing. Right? It's not something we are meant to openly admit that we experience, even though, let's face it, we all do experience it sometimes for all sorts of reasons. Mel believes that jealousy is simply *blocked desire*. When it bubbles within us, we shouldn't ignore it, but rather tune in to it as it might be giving us clues and directions about where we want to go in life.

The thing about jealousy is that you can't be jealous of something you don't desire. I will never be jealous of someone who has completed an Ironman, or of someone who has bought a house in Bali, as these are not things that interest me.

Jealousy can be our subconscious trying to tell us something important. We just need to listen. When someone does accomplish something that causes jealousy to arise, I need to pay attention to that and ask myself questions:

Why am I jealous of him/her/them?

What have they done to evoke that emotion in me?

I call this my 'jealousy compass'.

I challenge myself to not run away from jealousy. Instead, I acknowledge it. Sit with it. Explore it. It is bloody hard, but it can be enlightening. What we *don't* want to do is use jealousy to fuel toxic negativity or it will consume us. Instead, use it to motivate you, to set goals and chase ambitions. It can give us the impetus to move outside our comfort zone and take on new challenges, maybe ones we hadn't considered before.

Self-awareness is the key to understanding what jealousy is – and to thinking about how it shows up in each of us. Then at least we know to look out for it. I can be guilty of giving out or bitching when jealousy comes knocking on my door. How many of you are like me? In some, it can show up and affect their mood. For others, it can fuel suspicion and doubt.

Jealousy can give you direction on where you want to go, like a compass. It can help you to figure out what you want in life. Do you know what you truly want? And are you able to detach yourself from what you don't want? It's about allowing yourself permission to feel jealousy, but to observe it and tune in to it, and then make positive decisions to move forward on a new path.

A good place to start is to write down who and what you are jealous of, and then use those insights to create goals and an action plan for yourself.

18. Challenge the fear

'Each of us must confront our own fears,
must come face to face with them. How we
handle our fears will determine where we go
with the rest of our lives. To experience
adventure or to be limited by the fear of it'
— Judy Blume

Fear is a perfectly normal, not to mention vital, response that we all experience. If we didn't have fear we wouldn't be able to protect ourselves from threats. However, we should try not to let everyday fears hold us back as they tend to be more mental obstacles that limit our actions and decisions, and prevent us from making progress in our lives. They throw up fears of failure, vulnerability and commitment, and present us with states of being that we just don't want to occupy.

However, putting yourself in a position to try new challenges, opportunities and experiences can enrich your life in ways that staying safely in your comfort zone can never do. Imagine you could see all of the wonders of the world from one spot but the only way to see them is to cross a rope bridge. Imagine you would have all the safety harnesses and apparel there is, but it's still going to be daunting to cross that bridge. Would you go?

A lot of us might stay on the safe side, content with photos and retellings of the amazing wonders personally witnessed by others. We are so afraid of what might happen that we remain on the safe side without taking the opportunity to see something spectacular.

It's not that the people who choose to cross the bridge don't feel the fear. They do. Some of them will hide it, seem brash and confident, and cross quickly. Some will take it very slow, step by step, checking their safety gear over and over again, until they reach the other side. If you'd prefer to stay in the safe zone, that's understandable and maybe you're not ready, but why don't you think about whether you could choose the latter option? Why not take small steps, so small that the other side is not even in view, but you get closer to it with each move forward?

In Susan Jeffers' bestselling book *Feel the Fear and Do It Anyway* she says that the only way to get rid of the fear of something is to go ahead and do it. When making a lifestyle change of any kind, we should visualize that bridge. Some will bounce across the bridge without a harness, others are more cautious, but however you choose to get to the other side, you still reach the ultimate goal. Your approach, your process, is individual to you.

Jeffers maintains that there are five truths about fear:

- **Truth no. 1: The fear will never go away as long as you continue to grow**
  As long as you continue to take new risks or be confronted with new challenges in pursuit of your

goals, you're going to experience fear. You can't wait for the fear to go away to take the next step. If you're constantly saying 'When I lose some weight, then I'll join that running club', you're always going to lose. Why not just join the running club? Because otherwise you might find you put it off indefinitely.

- **Truth no. 2: The only way to get rid of the fear of doing something is to go out and do it**
  You can defeat your fear of a situation by confronting it. You join the running club, and yeah, you walked for a little bit, but not as much as you expected, and you had good fun chatting to the other members of the group. The next week, you ran a bit more, and the next week a bit more. Once you feel the fear and know that you can handle it, the fear subsides.

- **Truth no. 3: The only way to feel better about myself is to go out and do it**
  Once you feel better about yourself and know that you're capable, you might find your fear lessens and you become more confident. When you've finally mastered something and the fear disappears, it will feel so good that you want to challenge yourself and push yourself to find something new to accomplish. But then the fear creeps in again as you prepare for your next challenge. You're running

5km easily with the running club, and you've decided to push yourself and enter a race. The fear starts creeping in. *What if I'm last? What if I get a cramp? Will everyone be looking at me and judging my technique?*

- **Truth no. 4: Not only am I going to experience fear whenever I'm on unfamiliar territory, but so will everyone else**
  You may think that you are the only one who has this fear. But most people have similar feelings of fear and anxiety. It is not a feeling that is reserved for you alone, it is universal. You realize that everyone is nervous about the race, and has their own concerns, but you all support and encourage each other when you're warming up and at the starting line.

- **Truth no. 5: Pushing through fear is less frightening than living with the underlying fear that comes from a feeling of helplessness**
  Facing a new situation will always induce feelings of fear. But if you successfully push through it, you develop a sense of achievement that improves your confidence. You feel more capable of handling any curveballs that life may throw at you. You successfully complete the 5km race and feel elated. You celebrate with your running group and you're more determined than ever to move on to the next challenge.

229

Honestly, the fear never goes away for most of us. But as you can hopefully see from the above, it's not necessarily a bad thing. Even now, especially in the career I'm in, and years after starting out, I still feel the fear. Whether I'm about to stand up in front of a group and deliver a keynote speech or whether I'm about to go live on TV and I hear the words, 'And we're live in 3 . . . 2 . . . 1,' my fear is palpable. Sweating, dry mouth, tension across my shoulders, butterflies in my belly, the works. But once I get into the zone, I start to gain confidence and relax. I remind myself I can do tough things. The fear dissipates, and I am so proud once I'm done. I'm even looking forward to the next time!

While it is natural for me to feel fear, I actively try not to let it stop me. I have learned to lean in to the fear and reframe it positively in my mind. I'm feeling fear because I want it to work out, I want to do a good job, because I care about what I'm doing. If I wait for the fear to subside, I'll never do anything. If you just go for it, you prove to yourself that you can do it, *despite* the fear. You are capable, you are ready, you are strong – so just go for it!

Allow yourself to be vulnerable

'Vulnerability is not winning or losing; it's
having the courage to show up and be seen when
we have no control over the outcome'
– Brené Brown

I want to touch on vulnerability in the context of fear, as often it is the fear of being vulnerable that can prevent us from taking an opportunity or embarking on a new challenge. Facing our fear is challenging because we need to be open to be vulnerable, which is often an uncomfortable feeling for us all. It makes us feel unstable, or we sense a loss of control.

Even from the tender age of five, when I first began playing camogie, I was learning about challenge and how to step out of my comfort zone. Sport taught me that being vulnerable is part of life, even before I knew the word, and it taught me how to push through the fear. When you play sport, you learn that sometimes you let yourself and others down, but that you can move on and learn from it. It teaches you that those mistakes on the pitch can't be helped, but letting the team down in other ways, like not turning up for matches or training, *can* be helped. You learn what you can control and what you cannot.

Write down the things you would do in your life if fear wasn't an obstacle

In Byron Katie's book *Loving What Is*, one of the questions she asks is 'What would you be doing right now if you didn't have fear?'

What would you be doing if you didn't have that fear?

Let's say you would love to go travelling solo – you have a deep urge to experience the world your way, on your terms. You want to walk the Great Wall of China, you want to climb Machu Picchu, you want to dip your toes in the warm waters of the Indian Ocean.

That's the dream, but in truth you're too fearful and feel too vulnerable to even go away for a weekend in Ireland by yourself. So that's where you start. Start anywhere. But you must start. The emotions you'll feel, the racing heartbeat, the profuse sweating (oh, how I recognize the sweating), that will all come with the first time you raise a finger and say 'table for one'.

It will fade away once the reward comes i.e. following through and sitting there eating alone. Sure, you might feel vulnerable the first time. Making your order may feel awkward. You might tell yourself that you were wrong to do this because it feels so uncomfortable, right before you bury your head in your phone.

But do you believe that the same level of discomfort will continue if you have a meal out alone every week? You know it will fade and you will get used to eating on your own, watching the people around you, relaxing in your own company, without the phone. It might even become something you look forward to doing.

This is the same across the board with all the things we want, the things that sit in the opposite space from where we are now. Sometimes they are merely a few steps away. But taking even one step out of your comfort zone can feel like you are trying to leap over a deep chasm. Everything new requires us to feel a level of discomfort and vulnerability.

I experienced this when I took up boxing. I always remember watching the girl at the punchbag to my left. She was absolutely smashing it and I felt so inept, vulnerable and out of my comfort zone. Here I was, an All-Stars camogie champion, struggling to get to grips with the basics. But I reframed it in my mind. I tried to remember that she was once where I was, feeling the fear, but she was still there because she knew it was the only way to learn and grow.

Feeling vulnerability around people who can do better than us is an uncomfortable place to be. It would be so easy to just give up, there and then. But now I see her as my guide to growth. I'm not in her league – yet! – but I show up and I see myself improving every week, and it makes me feel good about myself.

The discomfort of feeling vulnerable often makes us question whether we can make bigger changes in our lives. Putting myself out there as a broadcaster made me feel immensely vulnerable. I was so worried about what people would think of me. Would they think that I was getting ahead of myself? But I had to ask myself what was the risk and what was the reward?

For me to fulfil my goals in life, I knew I had to say yes to the opportunity. This has led to more opportunities, and now

I'm presenting my own health and well-being show, *Super-charged with Anna Geary*, on RTÉ Radio 1. I am immensely proud of the show as it deals with important health concerns and issues, with a wide range of guests, from experts to ordinary people with real-life 'lived' experiences.

Don't be afraid to fail

'Don't be afraid to fail, be afraid not to try'
— Michael Jordan

It is completely normal when experiencing something new to question your ability to do it.

Holding back in life can operate as a form of protection mechanism, the thought process being *If I don't give everything of myself and I come up short, then I can choose to believe it was because I didn't fully apply myself.* To repeat: there is a vulnerability in giving 100 per cent of yourself to a goal. If it doesn't work out, you must face the fact that you weren't good enough at the time. Failure. The fear of failure can be crippling. It can cause us to fall into a state of inertia and, therefore, we stay the same, we don't move forward.

Failing can look different in different people. In some, it can be a reluctance to try something or take on a challenge. In others, it can look like self-sabotage, where they procrastinate until the opportunity passes them by, or they give up halfway through. It can also be a sign of a lack of self-confidence – *I'm not flexible enough to do yoga, so I won't.* It can also look like perfectionism, when someone will only do something if they know they can do it well, but won't try anything else. Failure comes in many forms and having to face up to failure can be a tricky thing. But we can't allow fear to stop us progressing in life and achieving our goals.

There is value in failing. Failure leaves clues. It can show us where we need to improve, it can highlight problems that we can find solutions for, it can force us into rethinking strategies to make them more effective in the long run. We can embrace it as a learning experience and try again. We need to rewire our mindset to see that failure is not the opposite of success; in fact, it is essential so that success can eventually follow. As Michael Jordan, one of the greatest athletes of all time, famously admitted, 'I've missed more than 9,000 shots in my career. I've lost almost 300 games. Twenty-six times I've been trusted to take the game-winning shot and missed. I've failed over and over and over again in my life. And that is why I succeed.' You won't know unless you attempt the shot.

Every time I played camogie, I made mistakes and had setbacks and challenging moments. But I learned from them and came back stronger. As captain, I had a responsibility to address things that weren't working and we embraced the idea of 'what gets measured gets managed'. If something wasn't working in the team or during a game, we asked why it didn't work, and we looked at tweaking and improving things. We didn't approach it as a failure, we approached it as a learning experience.

Our mantra was *Fail = first attempt in learning*. First, we needed to learn to accept the mistake, then we figured out how to work through it. Sometimes this is easier said than done and I know that better than anyone. In the world of sport, failure can often mean losing a match due to an error you made and you have to own that. It is a great life skill to learn, but also one of the most difficult.

Moving on from failure

Even in my personal life, I have struggled to take my own advice. When it comes to moving on from failure, I found it difficult. I remember in my final year of my business degree at the University of Limerick, I had razor-sharp focus going into my final exam. I had studied and prepared, and refused to be distracted from nailing this exam. It was my favourite module, and I wanted to get a great mark. I knew I could, I had everything I needed to ace it: the knowledge, the focus and the interest.

I went into the exam with that same attitude and I made the decision to focus only on the paper, blocking out all the nervous chatter from fellow students on the way in. I kept my head down for the whole exam – I just wanted to get the information inside my head down on to the paper as quickly and efficiently as possible. I had two and a half hours, three essays. I had the exam mapped out, I had timed this in my study sessions. I knew what I was doing. Just as I started into the third question, I was suddenly shocked by the voice of the examiner saying loudly, 'Ten minutes left.' And when I looked up, there in front of me, right in my eyeline, in huge black letters, was a sign saying THIS EXAM IS TWO HOURS.

It's a complete understatement to say that I panicked. I felt as though my stomach hit the floor and I desperately drew spider diagrams (you know the ones!) to jot down as much as I could for the third question, but I knew deep down my grade would suffer. All of my studying flew out of the window because of one simple reason: I failed to look up. I didn't take a minute to look around, to assess my environment. That small detail, which was entirely in my control, that decision to not be present, to not look around, impacted my final result. The frustration of one small, seemingly trivial mistake was hard to shake off, but it taught me a valuable lesson: always be prepared, always be observant – the smallest details matter.

Focus on the comeback, not the setback

Think about book and film plots. They always contain challenges and setbacks. These are the devices that give the storylines depth and draw us in. We want to see how things turn out, how the stories are resolved. How boring would the plot be if there were no twists and turns along the way? When it comes to the storyline of your own life, focus your energy on the comeback, not the setback. The comeback you can control; the setback is often beyond your control.

Control the controllables

The Swiss psychoanalyst Carl Jung said that when it comes to resilience, 'You are not what happened to you, you are who you choose to become.' So, it is not so much about what you experience, it is more about how you choose to react to and deal with it. That is what is within your control.

Control the controllables was something I learned from sport. You cannot have control if the referee gives an important score to the opposition (even if you believe it was in error), but you can control how you respond to it, and subsequently come back from it.

Next time you face an unexpected plot twist in your life, ask yourself, 'What's in my control?' and go from there.

Anna Wintour, *Vogue*'s illustrious editor-in-chief, once said that everyone should be 'fired at least once in their career' as it's 'a great learning experience'. In the early days of her career, she was let go from her job as junior fashion editor at *Harper's Bazaar* because her fashion shoots were considered too edgy. Anna had dropped out of college and taken a huge risk on a training programme that led to this job, and now it seemed it was all crashing down around her. Although the dismissal hurt and she was thrown off the course she believed she was on, with hindsight she says it was a catalyst for how successful she is today. She maintains that 'It's important to have setbacks because that is the reality of life.'

This is the thing . . . life happens. Sometimes, even with all your best behaviour, preparation and intentions, things just don't work out, and you have a setback or a failure. But I can safely say that it doesn't mean anything much, not in the long run. Those times when it feels like we are finished – we never are. I got over my bad exam, my lost matches, my job rejection, and still progressed to where I am now. We always need to hop back on the wagon and go again.

As babies, to learn to walk we have to fall. And later, as kids learning to ride bikes and turn cartwheels, we still have to fall. And as adults, we will experience falls too. We must experience the setback and live through the turmoil to reach even ground again. No journey is easy all the way. And sometimes the things that seem like the worst news ever – the exam fail, the break-up, the number on the scales going up instead of down – you need to accept that those things happen, and that these are the things that end up driving you to a better place than where you started. Detach failure from the negative emotions that often accompany it and take it as a chance to reflect and reset.

So how do we cope with failure? What techniques can we learn to make failure bearable and turn it into an opportunity for growth and learning?

- Allow yourself to feel upset, frustrated and disappointed, don't push those feelings away. Accept your humanity in those moments. Crawl under your duvet and cry your eyes out. Don't attempt to dissect the situation while you feel emotional. Wait and do that later.
- Adopt a growth mindset and ask yourself what steps you can take next time to avoid this happening again. Analyse and reflect on what went wrong and reflect on what you can do next time. Find the positives in the experience and focus on them.
- Be compassionate to yourself. What would you say to a relative or a friend if they were in the same circumstances? You probably wouldn't be berating them as hard as you are berating yourself. Try to avoid negative self-talk.
- Confide in family and friends, don't keep failures to yourself. Sometimes talking about it to another person can make you see it in a different light, and help you reframe your failure in your head, provide a sense of perspective and hopefully give you the support you need to try again.
- Think about the failure as an opportunity to rethink your priorities and goals.
- Persevere! Remember, Rome wasn't built in a day. The failure has brought you closer to your goal because you had the courage to put yourself out there.

Epic fails

We have been conditioned to look at failure in a negative light, something to be embarrassed about. We tend not to want to speak about the times we may have failed. Throughout this book I am trying to help you to understand that failures are part and parcel of life. Failures are not to be feared or avoided. They are not weaknesses. *Epic fails* is a tool I use to help reframe attitudes towards failure.

What is an epic fail? It's a time or experience in your life that you were sure would work out and it didn't, even though you really wanted it at the time. You thought it was exactly what you wanted and were so disappointed when it didn't go to plan.

You got let go from a job
You left a long-term relationship
You didn't get your first-choice college course
You didn't make a team squad

But, looking back, you realize that it was a brilliant thing to happen and ended up having a positive effect on your life. For example, maybe you lost a job and that was the catalyst for setting up your own business, or maybe the end of a relationship forced you back on to the dating scene and you met someone far more suited to you.

Write down your epic fails. Remember how you felt and consciously recognize that it happened for good reason.

The next time you experience an epic fail you might embrace it and not allow it to affect you the same way. Remember, failures are feedback – and they can give you insights into what you actually want. You just need to tune in to them.

Sometimes things fall apart so that better things can fall together.

19. Building your resilience

'The greatest glory in living lies not in never falling,
but in rising every time we fall'
— Nelson Mandela

There is no doubt that challenges in our life test our resilience. Adverse situations arise, we can fail at times, we can be pushed to our limits personally and professionally, but when it comes to building resilience, the thing to remember is that it's not about what happens to you, it's how you respond and learn from it. Indeed, it's important to remember this when you hear the word bandied about: resilience isn't some magical thing that some people are born with while others have very little. Once you understand that resilience is a mindset – a way of responding to life's challenges – then you can set out to develop resilience in yourself. That is liberating.

One of my all-time favourite books is *What I Know For Sure* by Oprah Winfrey. In it she says:

One of my greatest lessons has been to fully understand that what looks like a dark patch in the quest for success is the universe pointing you in a new direction. Anything can be a miracle, a blessing, an opportunity if you choose to see it that way.

I always think of this quote when I reflect on my retirement from the Cork camogie team in 2015. I didn't leave camogie altogether at that stage, I wasn't ready for that step yet, and so I still played with my home club, Milford. But my retirement from Intercounty camogie was one of the single most difficult decisions I had to make on my own.

I couldn't discuss it with my close circle as I knew they would say I should stay. After all, we were the reigning All-Ireland Champions and had a great chance of retaining our title. I had been the captain of that All-Ireland winning team and I was still in my prime at twenty-seven. But I knew, deep down, something was niggling away at me. I felt unsettled.

That winter, I was nursing a cracked shin injury and I missed the League campaign. I had gone back to qualify as an executive and performance coach at the same time, and so I was forced to face up to tough questions about my life, including what my life would be like after camogie.

I knew I had to make a huge life decision, and I wanted to control the narrative. I wanted to announce it formally, that I was planning to move to Dublin to focus on a new career, and I didn't want to make a half-commitment to the Cork team, missing training sessions, only being around at the weekends. I'm someone who likes to fully commit, and if I couldn't do that, it wouldn't be fair on my teammates or myself.

I can't say I was 100 per cent sure of my decision, but I was sure enough to make the leap of faith. I was lucky enough to get sound advice and support from Marty Morrissey, and he arranged for us to do a quick piece to camera on the RTÉ *Six One News*. I didn't think my retirement announcement was newsworthy until it aired and my phone went into meltdown. I got so many messages questioning my reasoning, as I expected – I was too young, I was coming off the back of being the captain of the All-Ireland winning team the year before, I was at the pinnacle of my career.

I knew there was never going to be a good time to leave, camogie was such a huge part of my identity and my life. Everything was dictated by sport: my relationships, my friends, my career. All of these were influenced by my commitment to the Cork team and I didn't regret one minute of it. But it was time to step back. I was on a new path, and I didn't quite know where it started or where it would lead me to. Everything was unfamiliar and daunting, and at the time I didn't know who I was without camogie.

Steering your own ship

Within a few months, I'd left my job and moved to Dublin. That September, not long after stepping away from the Cork set-up, I was asked to get involved in the punditry with RTÉ for the All-Ireland Finals. I did feel a pang of envy as the teams ran out on to the pitch, but I also felt a sense of fulfilment that I was where I wanted to be at that moment in time. It all sounds so simple and straightforward, but it wasn't. It was full of self-doubt, dead ends and anxiety, but it taught me how to have faith in myself and my choices. How to be resilient and persevere. And I'm so glad I did.

It might sound dramatic (I am a little dramatic), but there is a quote from one of my favourite poems, 'Invictus', that resonates with me: 'I am the master of my fate, I am the captain of my soul.' It's hands-down my favourite quote and one that I have almost had tattooed on my body twice (on both occasions I bolted from the tattoo shop – yes, I chickened out!). I find that quote to be powerful because it explains to me how my life can be viewed in two ways: as a life that dictates to me, or one that I can dictate. The captain of a ship has no idea what storms or squalls are ahead, but he is the one who steers the ship to safety when it runs into trouble. This is resilience, it's in the power behind trusting yourself to steer your own ship and building the skills to deal with issues your way, when they arise.

I have always admired my mam and the way in which she backs herself in her decision-making. Her process involves mulling it over quietly and then, once she makes up her mind, that's it. No second-guessing herself. She is resilient and doesn't look to blame others if she makes the wrong decision. That's the most impressive part. The resilience she possesses enables her to recover quickly should she make the wrong decision. She has always had the capacity to deal with challenging situations.

Whenever I have a tough decision to make, Mam is one of the first people I will call to chat things through. She is rational, yet empathetic. She's a great listener and is both practical and pragmatic. She has instilled in me the courage of conviction to just go for things, and if they go wrong, you can always fix them. She is a great sounding board too. I am an overthinker by nature, while she doesn't believe in wasting time and energy dwelling on and rehashing details. Her attitude is, make the decision and then it's on to the next one. I am *trying* to adopt that outlook more in my life, and in the meantime, having someone like that in my corner is something I'm very grateful for.

Tips to help build your resilience:

You might find you are resilient in the face of one challenge but struggle with another. It's always good to learn how to build your resilience through a strengths-based approach to overcoming challenges, like we've covered in earlier chapters. Here are some ideas:

- **Develop your self-regulation skills** – challenging times inevitably cause anxiety and stress so it's worthwhile trying some stress-reduction techniques such as breathing exercises (like the example below), and mindfulness apps (like the *Calm* app).
- **Acquire new coping skills** – journalling, reframing thoughts, exercising, improving diet and sleep hygiene can often help you feel more in control of a situation.
- **Put in place a strong support system** – talking to people who love and value you will always help you when things are tough.
- **Know your strengths** – tap into your strengths to help you through adverse times.

Sixty seconds of breathing

It all comes back to the breath when you're feeling overwhelmed and anxious. Deep breathing exercises allow your throat muscles to contract and expand your lungs.

Find a quiet, comfortable space where you can lie or sit down. Close your eyes. Breathe in slowly through your nose, fully expanding your abdomen as you fill your lungs with air. Then exhale slowly through your mouth.

Try extending your exhales, making them longer than your inhales. This will help slow your heart rate. Inhale for four seconds and exhale for six seconds. Repeat six times.

20. Tactics board for challenge

'Being challenged in life is inevitable,
being defeated is optional'
— Roger Crawford

We can be sure that we will always face challenges in our life. It's how we learn to deal with these challenges that's the most important thing. We can either shut ourselves off to growth and learning, or we can embrace challenges as opportunities — opportunities to live fulfilled, contented lives. I know which option I have chosen!

Anna's take-home points

- **Adopt a growth mindset** – don't feel threatened by change and reframe challenges as opportunities. There is so much to learn in life, so take advantage of everything it has to offer and see where it takes you.
- **Step out of your comfort zone** – they say a change is as good as a rest, so start making small, gradual

changes in your daily life that benefit you and bring you closer to achieving your goals.

- **Give saying yes a go** – have the courage and conviction to do what you really want to do.
- **Confront your fears** – and by doing so, you make them smaller and less daunting, leaving you the space to fully embrace any challenge that comes your way.
- **Know that it's okay to be vulnerable** – that's how we know we are stepping out of our comfort zone.
- **Reframe failure as progress** – remind yourself that you are learning from your mistakes and not failing.
- **Build your resilience** – it will help you get through tough challenges that you may face over the course of your lifetime.

Read

Mindset: The New Psychology of Success – Carol Dweck
Feel the Fear and Do It Anyway – Susan Jeffers
Loving What Is – Byron Katie
What I Know For Sure – Oprah Winfrey
Daring Greatly – Brené Brown
Awaken the Giant Within – Tony Robbins
Courage is Calling – Ryan Holiday

Listen

Calm app
Headspace app

250

How to Fail podcast – Elizabeth Day
The Diary of a CEO podcast – Steven Bartlett
Unspoken podcast – Clodagh Campbell
'Better Days are Coming' – Dermot Kennedy
'Fight Song' – Rachel Platten
'Stronger' – Kelly Clarkson

Watch

The Last Dance
Invictus
Friday Night Lights
You've Got Mail
The River Wild

Challenge – my personal tactics board

....

....

....

....

....

....

....

....

....

....

....

PART FIVE

Game Plan for Kindness

21. Kindness is powerful

'Wherever there is a human being,
there is an opportunity for a kindness'
— Lucius Annaeus Seneca

Be kind. You see those words a lot – *Be Kind!* – in pink swirly font emblazoned on T-shirts, notebooks, posters and other paraphernalia. Often to the extent that the words seem to lose all sense of meaning. But we shouldn't forget what kindness means and the impact it can have in both our own lives and the lives of people around us.

Kindness is underestimated. It has such an important place in the world, and it's something that we should never lose sight of in the face of challenges and adversity. The truth is that kindness is a powerful force that can bring joy, love and happiness to people.

Like everything else in this book, kindness is a practice. I suppose for me when I think about kindness, it's so much more than being nice. It's about being available as a friend, as a daughter, as a partner. It's giving time, support, care, and showing compassion to others, whether we know them or not. Kindness isn't always convenient, it doesn't tie in neatly with our plans, but when we practise kindness, or receive kindness, the benefits are huge.

Physiologically, kindness positively impacts our brains. In fact, being kind is proven to stimulate the release of hormones like serotonin (regulates mood), oxytocin (increases social bonding), dopamine (makes you feel good) and endorphins (relieve pain and stress). These hormones are responsible for us feeling satisfaction, pleasure and improved well-being. So, approaching life with an attitude of kindness is a proven antidote to pain, stress and anxiety.

Kindness is about the small stuff

Practising kindness doesn't mean that we live our lives as beacons of charitable perfection. And it doesn't mean that we won't get upset, annoyed and frustrated. Kindness is not about making grand gestures. It's often the small, sometimes fleeting moments where kindness is extended that can mean the most.

I'll never forget the kindness that people showed to both me and my family when my dad sadly passed away. People were so thoughtful. They drove from all corners of the country to see how I was doing, they sent meaningful cards, they checked in on my mam, they made long journeys to my dad's funeral. They went to such lengths to make sure I knew that they were thinking of me and my family. To me, their kindness had real impact. They went out of their way – put their own plans and lives aside – to console and comfort me. I will always be grateful for their support and compassion.

And so, to me, kindness means that you can be a better friend, a better partner, a better parent, a better colleague, and a better version of yourself. And that's the most important thing. We can build kindness into our lives as part of our new lifestyle. But we need to practise being kind to others *and* to ourselves.

22. The hardest kindness

'We can't practise compassion with other
people if we can't treat ourselves kindly'
— Brené Brown

Often, when we think of being kind, we are thinking of how we can be kind to others. But we can't be truly kind to others until we know how to be kind to ourselves. Self-kindness means to be compassionate to ourselves and ties in with the concept of self-acceptance and self-compassion we discussed in Part One.

If there's any type of kindness that needs to be practised, it's this one, as it does not come naturally to us. When something goes wrong, if we face adversity and we fail, self-kindness is often the first thing to desert us. We berate ourselves, beat ourselves up, and for what? So that we can feel even worse than we already do?

While I am in favour of acknowledging shortcomings, owning mistakes and admitting errors when things go pear-shaped or don't work out in our lives, long before we look for the lessons and the learnings, we need to practise internal kindness. No one deliberately goes out to make a mistake or a wrong decision or to underperform. It just happens – but tearing yourself down isn't going to rectify it. You don't learn anything from that, except perhaps a sense of reluctance to try again in the future.

If we show kindness to ourselves, we avail of so many positive consequences that make it much easier to pick ourselves up after a fall: emotional intelligence, resilience, happiness, positivity, connectedness with others. If we don't, the reality is that we are likely to be our own worst critics, riddled with anxiety, and set ourselves up for repeated knocks in life. I have already given you tips on how to be more compassionate to yourself in Part One, by reframing negative self-talk, banishing negative thoughts and embracing yourself for who you really are. Now I want you to take this compassion and practise it in your daily life by showing kindness to yourself.

Progress not perfection

'If I waited for perfection, I would never write a word'
– Margaret Atwood

Wouldn't it be great to be perfect? Sadly, this is a state that is impossible to achieve, but we are widely led to believe that it can be attainable. We chase it. We crave it. We obsess about it. There is a belief that if we live a perfect life, look perfect, act perfect, have perfect jobs, houses, careers and families, then we will be enough. We will feel like we belong, and we will feel loved.

261

We live in a society that presents us with perfect images and it can do massive damage to our sense of self-worth. With all the filters and Photoshop apps, and images of airbrushed perfection everywhere we look, it can feel like we are the only ones who aren't living the perfect life.

So, what happens? We buy into it and switch on the filters ourselves. How many of us have used those perfect skin filters on our Instagram (hello, Paris filter)? My hand is definitely raised! How many of us have presented the best moments of our lives while carefully leaving out the worst parts of our day?

Since I was young, I have been preoccupied with the idea of being perfect, and even now, though my logical adult brain knows perfection is impossible, I still sometimes measure myself against unrealistic standards. I have admitted there were times I didn't even want to try something, because I didn't know if I could do it, and I felt as though anything less than perfect was pointless.

I turned down the opportunity of playing in a charity golf tournament with some amazing people a few years ago because I feared I would make a show of myself. Even earlier than that, aged fourteen in Irish college, I remember pretending I had sprained my hand to avoid playing volleyball because I simply didn't know how to play. If I did anything, I wanted to be perfect at it. Have you ever felt like this?

I do know this about myself: even though I challenge that thinking every single day, it's still a huge battle. Now at least I will try new things, and I will do things I am unfamiliar with or might not be good at. These days I buckle up, put my head down and go for it – most of the time. But understanding myself doesn't stop me from feeling how I feel.

This book is a great example. I have wanted to write this book for so long, but I wanted it to be perfect. I wanted it to be the best book I could possibly write. I added things in, took things out, moved things around, wrote and rewrote. Then I realized what I was doing and saw that if I wanted to share what I have learned over the course of my life, I have to risk this book being less than perfect. Because I am not perfect.

I have to let it go to print and cross my fingers that it does what I set out to achieve, which is to impart my advice, and hope it helps you for the better, that you get some joy and inspiration from it. I learned to enjoy the process and focus on the progress that I made. Every 100, then 1,000 words I wrote, I felt a sense of achievement and another step closer to my goal.

Things will never be perfect, we can never be perfect, life will never be perfect. We can't keep waiting for a day that will never come. We have to dive into what we want now. I suppose it's a matter of unlocking confidence, and to do that we need to understand what confidence is.

People say to me sometimes that they wish they had my confidence, and it always makes me laugh, because I constantly need to battle with my lack of confidence. But I think I know what they mean. I don't let my lack of self-belief in some circumstances stop me being the person – or striving to be the person – that I want to be. I suppose the confidence that people see in me, it's just my courage to give things a go, to take advantage of opportunities even when I'm not sure I can do them at the time. The more things I do, the more things I try, the easier it becomes to quieten those inner voices and outside critics, and just do the things I want to do. Maybe that's what they mean when they say confidence comes from within. In my case, it's a loud *shush* to my negative thoughts.

Likewise, I've learned to embrace the feelings of nerves, to reframe them and think of them as feelings of excitement and anticipation. Nerves show that your body and mind are building up to something. As I say to younger people all the time, if you are nervous about something, it's a good thing. It shows that what you are about to do matters and that you care about the outcome.

I suppose we could say that real confidence comes from a willingness to try when you don't know how it will turn out. Back in Irish college, I know now it was fear that stopped me trying volleyball. I identified as the 'sporty one' and to perform badly at a sport would have shaken my identity.

Think of the identity you like to present to the outside world, the descriptions you would like to have used about you so it seems like you're living a perfect life e.g. 'amazing friend', 'sporty', 'early riser', 'great craic', 'fantastic cook', 'ambitious', 'brilliant parent', 'perfect skin', 'stylish', and so on. Ask yourself what it would be like to detach from all these labels, to untether yourself from the image you try to present to the world. Who are you without the labels? Even if they are all positive and worthwhile, do they all align with your true self, your interests and your purpose? Basing your sense of self-worth on seeming perfect to others takes up a lot of time and energy that you could use to focus on what genuinely fulfils you.

By wanting to be perfect, we often engage in self-defeating thoughts that make it harder for us to progress, or even to have fun and enjoy ourselves. I want you to be kinder to yourself, to realize that you don't have to be the best at everything but rather to live your life to your best capabilities. Get the most you can out of each day. And you do this by focusing on your progress – what you have already achieved can motivate and inspire you. You will develop a greater sense of self-belief and it will give you the confidence to take on brilliant and exciting opportunities that may come your way.

Identifying perfectionist triggers

If you are susceptible to seeking perfection, there are possibly reoccurring triggers to look out for. To identify which areas you are striving for perfection in, notice the patterns around your behaviour anytime you focus on a particular area – maybe it's to do with your body, your career, your children.

Start with the end in mind and work backwards. Say you are berating yourself about your body. What happened that day? Think back. Did someone pass a comment, did you not prepare your lunch and so had to grab something on the go, did you miss a workout, did a dress no longer fit when you tried it on?

Identify the triggers and then, when they arise again, you will be aware that these are your triggers and be prepared for them.

Don't be a people-pleaser!

'When you say yes to others, make sure you aren't saying no to yourself'

– Paulo Coelho

There is a big difference between practising kindness and engaging in the unhealthy habit of people-pleasing. People-pleasing is when we continuously or almost chronically put other people's needs before our own and to the detriment of ourselves. Sometimes it's difficult to distinguish the fine line between being kind and being a people-pleaser. So how can we tell one from the other when on the outside they both manifest the same? The difference is how they feel to you on the inside.

We all people-please to some extent, and I don't know if we can ever completely eradicate people-pleasing from our lives. We say yes to things we would rather say no to, because we love the person asking or we genuinely want to help and so put ourselves second in a situation. I am no different.

I will go to see a film I'm not mad about seeing or watch a show because my husband loves it. I often compromise when I want to spend time with people I care about. I have also sat in restaurants and nodded to the waiter enthusiastically and given the thumbs-up mid-chew to a lukewarm, mediocre meal. I've told hairdressers and make-up artists they did a 'fab job' and have gone home to scrub their hard work off and redo it myself because it wasn't done how I like it. Those things are normal.

So, why do we people-please? I think women more than men are conditioned to behave in certain ways – *to be a good girl* – and so many of us go out of our way to make others feel comfortable and fulfil their needs, sometimes to the detriment of our own needs.

As a child I wanted to please my parents. I wanted to come home from school with good marks, I wanted to be good at my sport, and I liked the feeling of making my parents happy. I liked how their responses would make me feel: 'You're so good,' 'You're so reliable.' And with these positive responses from adults, I felt worthy of love and acceptance. In fairness to them, I could have done one tenth of what I achieved and they would still have been delighted and proud – the pressure never came from them, but I put myself under that pressure.

I did, for a long time, get into the habit of people-pleasing. I couldn't stand the thought of other people being upset with and disappointed in me. I didn't want to let them down, so I let me down.

One of the last times I remember people-pleasing was when I ended up going to an event I didn't want to go to, all because I couldn't put myself first. It is always such an honour to be invited to parties and events, and I love the glam and meeting people, but sometimes, for a myriad of reasons like work, family or health, it's not the right time to accept. This was one of those times. I was busy with work and I knew I had a big day scheduled for the day after the event that required a lot of preparation. But I agreed because my friend urged me to go with her.

On the day, my friend texted to say she wasn't feeling well and couldn't attend. I froze when I saw her message. It was too late for me to back out too. I didn't want to pull out last minute and let the outfit designer or the events team down, or come across as unreliable, so I went ahead. I remember sitting having my hair and make-up done and just wishing I could go home. My mind was on the work I should have been doing, not on the event. Then, to make matters worse, I remember arriving at the event and someone made a passive-aggressive remark about what I was wearing, and it knocked me. I felt vulnerable on my own and headed straight to the bathroom to regroup. At that moment I decided I wouldn't ever put myself in that situation again.

It was a stark reminder that my default is to people-please. I put my needs last because I didn't know how to deal with the bad feelings I got from letting people down. The fear of what they would think or say or feel was why I went. And the truth is it wouldn't have been a big deal if I hadn't gone. There would have been another time to wear the outfit and meet people. Where was that logical voice when I needed it?

When we people-please, it's often because we feel like we can't say no. But by saying yes, we open ourselves to negative feelings of frustration and resentment. Our choice is almost taken away from us because we are worried about causing someone else disappointment, making them angry, filling us with guilt.

When we show kindness to people, we do so out of our own choice, one that aligns with our values. This is the core of the matter: when we people-please we are not making the choice from the right place, we are not being kind because we want to – we are being kind because we are afraid of what will happen if we aren't. Kindness is when we do things because we really want to, because we care about the person and because we want to share. That's the kindness that we need in our life. The one that comes from our free will.

Understanding your motivation

If someone asks something of you, or you're placed in a situation where you're unsure of what to do for the best, ask yourself the following questions before deciding how to respond:

Why do I feel like it's my responsibility to make them feel good?
Why am I afraid of saying no?
Where does this fear come from?
Why am I afraid of disappointing this person?
Why do I think that I'll be rejected if I say no?

Self-care

'It is so important to take time for yourself and find
clarity. The most important relationship is the one
you have with yourself'

– Diane von Fürstenberg

Self-compassion is regarding yourself kindly, and self-care is treating yourself kindly. They are two different processes – thought and action. Self-care is taking care of yourself so that you can be healthy, you can be fit, you can do your job and you can be there for the people who are important to you. It's about looking after yourself so you can stay physically, mentally and emotionally well. It lessens stress and anxiety, decreases the chance of burnout, and allows you to feel more control in your life.

It's worth noting that there is a huge difference between self-care and self-indulgence. If you think being nice to yourself involves binge-watching an entire series on Netflix and eating your own body weight in ice cream, then you may not have fully grasped the essence of what self-care is. It's about wanting the best for your health and well-being because you care about yourself.

It's difficult to think about self-care when we live increasingly busy lives, but this ties in with what we spoke about in Part Three about the importance of changing up routines and habits, and prioritizing the important things in life. It might be helpful to develop a self-care plan when you are thinking about any lifestyle changes.

Self-care plan

Sit down and assess areas of your life that you feel might need a little more attention and care.

- Assess your needs. Make a list of the most important activities that you do every day. *Work, preparing meals, looking after your family, playing a sport, walking the dog . . .*
- Consider your stressors. What areas cause you most stress? How can you alleviate that stress? *The traffic on the commute to work, school run, the weekly shop? Cycle instead of drive? Can you share drop-offs with other parents, do an online food shop?*
- Devise a self-care strategy. Think of some activities that might help you feel better. *A massage, meeting a friend for a walk, reading before bed.*
- Schedule time to focus on your needs. Make your self-care a priority.

Self-care isn't selfish! If it affords you the chance to feel better in yourself, feel more refreshed and rejuvenated, then in turn you will show up as a better version of yourself in your life and in the lives of others. It helps you become a better parent, partner, friend, colleague, neighbour, sibling, carer. It's worth investing the time.

I've listed a few ideas for some acts of self-care that can boost your mood and improve your health. By incorporating one or all of these into your life, you may feel some positive benefits to your physical and emotional well-being.

- **Exercise** – there are so many benefits to exercise, including improved brain function, weight management, improved quality of sleep, improved heart and lung function, strengthening of bones, reduced feelings of stress and anxiety . . . need I go on?!
- **Diet** – we all know it's hard to change our diet. But start slowly and make gradual changes. I would suggest that you add in more fermented foods to your diet, like sauerkraut, probiotics and kombucha, to improve your gut microbiome. A healthy gut will boost your immunity levels and improve your digestion, brain and heart health too. Another thing I would suggest is to add more protein to your diet as it improves satiety levels and helps the growth of lean muscle mass, so think about incorporating more fish, eggs, lean meats, nuts and a range of peas and beans in your meals.
- **Vitamin D** – you might find it worthwhile to take Vitamin D supplements to boost your immunity levels during the winter months. It's worth chatting to your local pharmacist to see what they would advise.
- **Sleep** – good sleep hygiene is fundamental for our sense of well-being. Put your phone away at least an

hour before bed, read a good book instead, and try to get at least seven hours of sleep.

- **Getting out into nature** – this is just good for the soul. Take a walk with a friend or your partner in the park, by a river, in the woods, on the beach. Or go alone – it's a perfect opportunity to think things through and self-reflect.
- **Being sociable** – going out for a coffee, a few cocktails, dinner with friends, family or your partner can be so beneficial to your emotional well-being. It reinforces your connection with others.
- **The nice things** – if a manicure, massage or getting your hair done makes you feel better, and they are important to you, then make sure to schedule them in.

The friend audit

'Friendships between women, as any woman will
tell you, are built of a thousand small kindnesses . . .
swapped back and forth and over again'
– Michelle Obama

Friendships are there to nourish and sustain us. They are give and take – sometimes we will need the support of a friend and other times we are there to be a shoulder to cry on. Friendships are based on shared connections, values and experiences. We all have different types of friends in our lives. There are the ones you have fun with, the ones who you can chat to for hours, ones you go for walks with, the schoolfriends, the college gang, the work pals, the friends' wives, the social media friends . . . the list goes on. They're not all the same, and you're those kinds of friend to other people too.

And we know the difference between one kind of friend and another. We know – or we think we know – the friend who will drop it all and be there when the chips are down. But what about that friend who never remembers your birthday even though you always remember hers? The one who never sends a Christmas card or a housewarming card even though you never forget to send them to her? Sometimes we suddenly realize that the friend we thought we had isn't really there any more.

Visualizing your friendships

Think of your life like a solar system where you are the earth. Place the people in your life who love, accept and support you as close as the moon, and plot the others working outwards.

Think about the people who you want to limit your time with, those who don't make you feel good or those with toxic traits. Put them as far away as Neptune.

Create your boundaries and think of this visual representation when deciding where to spend your time and energy.

We all develop – at different rates and capacities – and so too do our friendships. Some pass the test of time, while others are there for whatever stage of your life you're in. When we stop and take a good look at our friendships, we may realize that some friends don't know us for who we are now. And that's okay, even though it might hurt at the time.

If you are continuously growing and evolving, then it's likely that they are too and maybe you are both going in different directions. You might have different interests or different goals, or be at different stages in your life. Maybe the friendship might take a backseat for now, only to gather momentum again when your lives realign.

I've learned two things in the year following my dad's death and suffering that incredibly intense loss. The first is that not everyone defines friendship in the same way that I do. I've also learned that I cannot hold other people accountable to the same standards that I set for myself when it comes to friendship. Those standards are based on my values, my priorities, and not everyone operates from the same value system, nor should they.

It's important to maintain and nurture our friendships if we genuinely want to stay emotionally connected. It's equally important to move away from the friendships that no longer serve us. Rather than questioning and filling ourselves with self-doubt, wondering what went wrong, if we did something to upset them – just let it go. There doesn't need to be drama or animosity. Just a parting of ways. It will be sad, but sometimes it's kinder to yourself in the long-term.

Common signs that you need to re-evaluate a friendship:

- You are not their priority. They don't make an effort to meet up or visit you. You always have to initiate contact. They might cancel on you regularly.
- You give more than you receive. In a friendship there may be times when one person needs to do more for the other. They, or you, might be going through a tough time. It's not always going to be a 50/50 split but there does need to be give and take. If you find you are always the one there for them, then that might cause friction and dissatisfaction.
- You don't connect in the same way. Connection is the bedrock of a friendship. If you no longer have things in common, the friendship may become strained.
- They don't celebrate your wins. Any successes you enjoy are reluctantly acknowledged, but when you do have setbacks they are dissected in far greater detail.

The friendship test

If you are worried about a friendship, and wondering if you should make the effort to maintain it or just cut loose, ask yourself the following questions:

Does their friendship bring you joy?
Do they support you through tough times?
Do they accept and love you for who you are?
Do they listen to you if you have a problem – or do they make it about them?
Do you actually want to be friends with them?

Remember: *Friends are the family we choose for ourselves.* They are there to lift us up, not to drag us down or drain us. It's impossible to remain friends with everyone in your life. By trying to do so you end up diluting the energy you have for your close few.

23. Loving yourself, imperfections and all

'Practising self-love means learning how to
trust ourselves, to treat ourselves with respect,
and to be kind and affectionate to ourselves'
— Brené Brown

When we think about love, we often think about it in relation to other people – generally, it's a feeling we reserve for the most special people in our life. We rarely think about love in terms of ourselves. The idea of learning to love yourself is inextricably tied up with self-acceptance, and I touched upon this concept of self-love in chapter 4.

You look after the people you love, you find time for them, you listen to them, you care about their well-being – all these things you should apply to yourself too. Being kind to yourself like you would any other person you care about is not selfish. It is how you love yourself. Don't think of self-care as making yourself a cup of tea or running yourself a hot bath. Think of self-care as having an active interest in what you are doing, where you are going in life, how you are feeling.

Think about the people you love most in the world. You probably don't like every single thing about them all of the time, do you? Some days, they will be awesome. Other days, they will irritate you intensely. But you would never say that you don't love them. When we love people, we love them, imperfections and all. We can recognize that humans are flawed, imperfect beings, but we love them all the same. And, likewise, the people who love us don't expect us to be perfect.

We put ourselves under huge pressure to be perfect, we hold ourselves up to impossible standards. Family and friends love us because of what we add to their lives, not because we have great eyebrows or got 600 points in our Leaving Cert ten years ago. When we make demands of ourselves to hit certain standards and to never fail, we miss out on the experience of having a good relationship with ourselves. We're too busy berating ourselves. Treat yourself like you would your best friend – with kindness and compassion.

Self-belief – have confidence in yourself

'Make the most of yourself,
for that is all there is of you'
– Ralph Waldo Emerson

The concepts of self-acceptance, self-compassion and self-belief are all linked. If you are compassionate to yourself, you are more likely to accept yourself for who you really are, and as a result you will have more confidence in your capabilities. You will have belief in yourself that you are good enough, and yes, you can take on a job, a task, a challenge.

Self-confidence is not a state of perpetual fearlessness, or never having any doubts, worries or regrets. Everyone carries worries and regrets, no matter how confident they are. Self-belief is a constant practice of self-acceptance – think of it like personal training for your heart and mind.

There have been times in my life when people have commented that they wish they had my confidence. I always laughed to myself, because there have been so many – too many – times when I've struggled with confidence. I couldn't accept myself as myself, and couldn't feel good about who I was, how I looked, or my capabilities as a sportsperson.

Remember the story I told you in chapter 2, about how I had to acknowledge my weaknesses and play to my strengths when I was moved out of my usual position in the Cork team? And how my self-belief was at an all-time low after the loss of the Final?

I went back to play with my club in Milford once the Intercounty season was over. On my first day back at training I felt like I was a ghost of my former self as I came out on to the pitch, where my club manager, Frankie, was waiting. Looking back now, it's obvious that I was negatively impacted by the changes and the loss. And he could see that. He said to me, 'Just go on out and play, Anna, just express yourself, just play the game you know and love.'

He trusted me and just let me play camogie. Getting that encouragement from him, and backing myself, helped me to rediscover my strengths as a player. I remembered why I played camogie, I remembered who I was as a player, my love for the game came back, and so did my self-belief and confidence. During that season with Milford, we won our first Senior Club title. We did it against the odds and it was a momentous achievement for the club and the wider community.

When I went back to play for my county the following season, I was back in the number-seven position. Getting back to wearing the number-seven jersey with Cork, in my favourite position, was testament to that renewed self-belief. I was made captain that year, in 2013. That same season we won the National League title and the Munster Championship.

In 2014, I was captain again and had the privilege of climbing the steps of the Hogan Stand to accept the O'Duffy Cup after winning the Senior Championship All-Ireland Final. Raising the cup felt like the most triumphant, amazing achievement. It was a dream come true and an accumulation of years of hard graft and perseverance. Accepting myself, my strengths, my flaws, showing compassion to myself and practising self-belief – they all helped get me to that Final.

For me, confidence comes from having the courage to *try*. And the more you try things, the more you back yourself in those situations, the more your self-confidence grows. True confidence has to come from within. It starts with self-acceptance and how you see yourself. It starts with being kind to yourself.

And never be afraid of nerves. Lean in to them. They are a signal that you care about what you are about to do. I don't know what type of person can start a new job, relationship or class without nerves. Nerves are natural when we are going into an uncertain and new situation. Your adrenaline is heightened, your heart is beating faster, you are mentally preparing yourself. Feeling the nerves and going ahead anyway is where confidence grows from.

Confidence booster – the Stanislavski System

This system was created by Konstantin Stanislavski, a Russian theatre director and actor. With the Stanislavski System, you focus on recalling experiences that showcased you working to your full capability. When you recall the accomplishment, you put yourself back inside the emotions of that experience. This will help you remember your power, your talents and capabilities, and build your self-confidence and self-belief.

Confidence is the willingness to try, even when you don't know how it's going to turn out. It's walking into a room and saying 'I am willing to give this a go'. Sometimes you will smash it, sometimes it won't go according to plan (I've been here lots of times), but the more you put yourself out there, the easier it gets. And the starting point for putting yourself out there is to treat yourself with respect and kindness.

24. Being kind to others

'No act of kindness,
no matter how small, is ever wasted'

– Aesop

Practising kindness is proven to inject a sense of positivity into your life and improves your self-esteem and sense of self-worth. Small acts of kindness, like gently freeing a butterfly out of the window, offering your place in the queue to the woman behind who only has one item, and being patient with the learner driver who has stalled three times at the green light, are all small, fleeting examples of acts of kindness that can positively impact your own mental health.

Practising kindness and showing empathy, compassion and understanding towards others makes them feel good and, by extension, we feel good. We're happy because we made someone else happy. In some small way, we have made an impact on someone else's life.

Whether it's a card in the post, a surprise bunch of flowers or a small gift that carries sentimental value, these little acts can have a disproportionately positive effect on someone. Something as simple as a timely, thoughtful message, call or even a hug can make a huge impression too. Have you ever got a text or a phone call from someone exactly when you needed it?

As Cork captain, or even as a senior player on any team, I was always aware of the younger players on the panel, encouraging them and helping them to feel included and comfortable. If they did something positive at training or tried something new, had a great performance in a match, or sometimes more importantly, if they didn't play well, a few words of support made a big difference. For you to take the time, to make a conscious effort, counts for a lot, just to let them know they're being acknowledged.

I remember going to an away match early in the season with some new players on the panel, so everyone was still getting to know each other. When I got on the bus, I noticed one of the younger players was sitting on her own so, without making a fuss, I asked if I could sit down beside her. She didn't say anything, she just smiled and moved over in the seat. I could tell that she was nervous because I'd been exactly where she was years before. She started to relax over the course of the journey. I got to know her better, who she was as a person, not just as a player. In any future exchanges we had after that she was a lot more confident to approach me for a chat, which was great. It was a small act but made a lasting impression.

Finally, there are times when you're just stumped. Maybe someone is dealing with challenges in their health, or going through some major life crisis, and you want to do something to show them your support but can't figure out what.

In those cases, don't get fixated on working out what you can do. Instead, ask this simple question: *What do you need from me today?* Giving another person the opportunity to ask for what they need is a powerful practical act of kindness.

Pay it forward

'Carry out a random act of kindness,
with no expectation of reward, safe in the knowledge
that one day someone might do the same for you'
– Princess Diana

As I mentioned in chapter 22, kindness is a choice that we make of our own free will. We see someone who needs to be shown kindness and we are happy to give them the kindness they need and deserve, with nothing in return for us – except for a feeling of warmth that we did something positive for someone else.

The pay-it-forward effect is simply where someone performs a single act of kindness, and this creates a chain reaction of kindness. The person who first receives the kindness pays it forward to someone else, and they pay it on to the next person, and so on. This creates a sense of connectedness and, when we are connected, we feel more supportive of and compassionate to others – whether friends, family or strangers.

Years ago, a friend of mine arranged for me to have a chat with someone she knew in the field I was looking to get a job in, to give me some advice and help me prepare for an inter-view. A while later, I did the same for someone else, because I knew how much it helped me when I was first starting out in my career.

Be the person who hands your parking ticket to the next car pulling in because there is an hour left on it, or the one who stops to help the man who fell over the kerb and has dropped his shopping. Don't be the person who walks by. Decide to live your life with kindness. You won't regret it.

Be kind with your words

'When words are both true and kind,
they can change the world'

– Buddha

Social media has elevated the level to which people can comment on the lives of others – hurtful comments can be made directly, anonymously and instantly. Commenting on other people isn't a new phenomenon, but with social media it's now so pervasive. The level of vitriol that we witness in the comments sections of Twitter, TikTok and Instagram is reaching new heights.

I'm not sure why we need to comment on others. Maybe it reflects dissatisfaction in our own lives, or we need to vent so we pick an easy target. But when we speak negatively about others, we are often in a negative headspace. Speaking kindly to someone makes you feel the opposite – it makes you feel good about yourself.

Can you frown and smile at the same time? Well, maybe you can, but it looks weird. Try it now, look in the mirror and attempt it. Essentially you have to choose a side – do you choose to practise behaviours that will foster either further positivity or negativity in your life? I'm not saying you will only ever be on one side, life doesn't work like that. It's only natural that everyone has good and bad days, and positive and negative moments within those days, but in general you will usually lean towards one. Then your energy becomes inextricably linked with that way of thinking.

Have you ever been bitching about someone and then when you say it out loud to someone else who doesn't agree with you, you don't know how to react? By verbalizing it, it becomes real, and you really understand the force of those words. Do you feel bad about yourself? Do you start to question yourself? Maybe it's a reality check that you are wasting energy talking negatively about someone when you could be channelling that energy in a more positive way.

If you have ever been ridiculed, belittled or devalued in person or online, then I get it. I understand that feeling. Many of us do in some way, which is a sad thing when you think about it. Even though we tell ourselves that cruelty comes from a place of pain, it doesn't make much difference to how it makes us feel and we will still question ourselves because of it.

No matter what we tell ourselves, cruel comments hurt. Careless comments can linger for years. They can be a catalyst to a life-long issue with yourself, long after the person has forgotten your name. You end up focusing on the perceived negative when you recall the comment, you feel the hurt again and again, and you feel bad about it. In worst-case scenarios, you may end up following fad diets, withdrawing from friends, losing self-confidence – essentially limiting your self-worth and the ability to progress in your life.

Once you say something, you can't unsay it

It's always important to think before we speak and to try to frame our words to others with as much kindness as possible. We don't know what someone is going through, and what we say and the way we say it can have an impact. For example, imagine you're out for dinner with a group of friends, and one of them orders a burger, and someone else comments, 'Oh my God, are you planning to eat all of that big, dirty burger?' They might say it as a joke, a flippant, throwaway comment, but it's loaded with judgement – and the recipient might feel self-conscious, be afraid to be seen eating and let it ruin their night out. Or the same thing could happen if someone was to comment negatively on what someone else was wearing. Why does it matter to them? Why should they judge someone else's choice of outfit? The more we train ourselves to not comment on someone else's personal preferences, the nicer we will all become.

I'm a first-time mum and I'm sure lots of women in the same position as me have found this, but announcing your pregnancy makes you fair game for people to give you 'help-ful' advice. This advice often seems to take a more negative slant on something which should be amazing and joyous. 'God, you'll never get your body back again,' 'You better sleep while you can,' 'Your nipples will be in bits,' 'Think it's bad now, wait until you go into labour' . . . I could go on. Pregnancy, childbirth, parenthood – they can all be overwhelming experiences so let's try to choose kindness when people are already in fragile states!

Before you say something to someone, think: *How would I feel if someone said this to me? Would I be happy? Hurt? Angry?* Think of the impact of what you say. This is so important that I'll repeat the title of this section: *Once you say something, you can't unsay it.*

Knowing when to filter out the trolls

When I was in my twenties, I would see comments made about photographs of me playing camogie. Anytime I saw references made to my body, particularly my muscular legs, I grew defensive and insecure, mostly the latter. A still image isn't always the most flattering when you are moving. It's called an action shot for a reason, as we are bending, twisting and turning in the heat of battle on the pitch. And let's not forget the game faces that go hand in hand with intense play – determined and often frowning or grimacing with gritted teeth as you tackle your opponent. But we are performing, not posing!

I'll admit that those comments often got into my head, and I would feel so self-conscious, when all I was doing was trying to be the very best at my sport. The critical commentary about my physical appearance and my personality continued when I appeared on sports programmes, or as a coach on *Ireland's Fittest Family*, or as a contestant on *Dancing with the Stars*.

By the time I appeared on *Dancing with the Stars*, I had become a bit savvier. I entrusted my close friend Paddy with my social media passwords. Every week after the show aired, he went through the comments, blocking or deleting any that were cruel. I didn't mind the constructive criticism, but the unnecessarily nasty comments were deleted. I knew, both from experience and understanding the concept of negativity bias, that I would focus more on the unpleasant comments rather than on the positive ones.

Asking Paddy to monitor my comments was the best thing I ever did. I never found out what the trolls thought of me, I never got to see the unkind insults that I know would have lingered in my mind. I was feeling vulnerable enough learning a new skill on a live show, and asking a friend to filter malicious comments meant that I really enjoyed the experience and wasn't afraid of the feedback. If you find yourself getting trolled online, take necessary steps. Thankfully, I don't come across it too often and for that I am grateful, but I am not naive enough to think that it doesn't exist.

Protect yourself

Imagine you had €86,400 in your bank account and someone stole €10. Would you get rid of the rest of the money – a sizeable €86,390? Of course you wouldn't. Because that money holds value, you can do so much with it.

There are 86,400 seconds in every day. If someone steals ten seconds of your day with a nasty comment, negative remark or confrontational email, take a moment and ask yourself, *Am I going to give them the remaining 86,390 seconds of my day?*

Showing kindness to yourself starts by protecting yourself, your mood and your energy. Your well-being is your responsibility. Don't give away that power.

Kind words can be inspirational

For any negative reactions I receive, I have found great comfort and support from the kindness shown to me by so many people. I truly appreciate every single kind reaction or comment, and in turn make the effort to pay that kindness forward, as you never know who may need it.

Shortly after the first *Dancing with the Stars* live show aired, I received an Instagram message from a woman whose daughter was a rower. She wanted to thank me for appearing on *Dancing with the Stars*. Her teenage daughter had quit rowing, despite a real love for it, because she was afraid of building too much muscle and didn't want to bulk up on her shoulders and look, in her words, 'masculine'. However, when her daughter watched me and saw my muscular body, she returned to rowing that week. My body, my muscles, had looked appealing to her daughter, and had helped ease her body anxiety.

That one kind message changed everything for me. I knew I couldn't let the idea of what people might think or say about me or my body stop me from doing my absolute best. What I was doing was a hugely positive thing, because I could use that platform for good, to be a role model of sorts for younger girls.

Now I wanted my muscles to be seen, for all those kids out there. I wanted them to see a woman who was proud of the body she had worked so hard on. I wasn't just there for me any more, I was representing athletes. The significance of being a sportswoman with a sportswoman's body was my renewed purpose on that show. The power of that woman's kind words gave me the confidence and incentive I needed. I went out on to the dance floor week after week and gave it my all.

25. Tactics board for kindness

'Be kind whenever possible. It is always possible'
— Dalai Lama

The value of kindness is immeasurable. If there's one practice we should incorporate into our lives daily, it's to be kind – to ourselves and to others. When we are kind, we feel better about ourselves and inject positivity into the lives of others, as well as our own. We can't control what anyone else does or says, but we do have control over our own thoughts and actions. We can't make anyone else kind, but that doesn't stop us from aiming to be kind to ourselves, to our family, to our friends and to strangers.

We can choose kindness. Even when it's not easy to do so.

Anna's take-home points

- Kindness starts with ourselves – make sure to prioritize self-care and self-compassion in your daily routine. Look after yourself and you can look after others.

- Being kind to yourself is remembering that you are not perfect, nor should you be. Your flaws, your failings, make you who you are, and people will love and support you regardless. Focus on your progress, not on always being perfect, and you will live a happier life.
- Remember, kindness is a choice that aligns with our values. If your choice is taken away from you because you are worried what will happen if you don't do something, it is not coming from a place of kindness but obligation.
- Practising acts of kindness, no matter how small, will help you feel connected to people you love and know, and to others in your wider community.
- Be kind with your words. Think before you speak or write something. Think about the place your words are coming from. Are they coming from a genuine place of compassion, concern, support or love? If they aren't, think twice. You never know the impact they will have on someone.

Read

Why Has Nobody Told Me This Before? – Dr Julie Smith
How to Win Friends and Influence People –Dale Carnegie
The Confidence Kit – Caroline Foran
The Boy, The Mole, The Fox and The Horse – Charlie Mackesy
Good Vibes, Good Life – Vex King
Joyrider – Angela Scanlon

Listen

Ready to be Real podcast – Síle Seoige
Owning It podcast – Caroline Foran
'Reach' – S Club 7

Watch

The Blind Side
The Shawshank Redemption
The Green Mile
The Lion King
Sweet Magnolias

Notes

Kindness – my personal tactics board

....

....

....

....

....

....

....

....

....

....

....

Final Thoughts

'We ask ourselves, "Who am I to be brilliant,
gorgeous, talented, fabulous?" Actually,
who are you not to be?'
– Marianne Williamson, *A Return to Love*

The wish I had when writing this book was to help you conquer your hang-ups, unlock your confidence and discover your purpose. To encourage you to take on new opportunities in order to achieve what you really want in life.

In a world where we are bombarded with images of perfection, it is sometimes easy to fall into a pit of despair – we're not good enough, we're not attractive enough, we're not successful enough, we're not skilled enough. But you don't need to be perfect – nobody is.

Is this a bad thing? Absolutely not. It is perfectly fine to be enough. To be happy and accepting of who you are and confident to go out and create the life you want to lead.

My hope is that by reading this book – whether you dip in and out of it when you have five minutes to spare, or read it all in one sitting – you have discovered new ways of finding out how you can become the most powerful version of yourself. That you have found methods and techniques that will show you how to embrace new opportunities, overcome challenges and incorporate elements of change into your daily life that impact you for the better.

I have always believed that making progress, no matter how small, how inconsequential it may seem, is better than making no progress at all. Doing something is always better than doing nothing. Because it means you are trying, you are moving forward, you are embracing life and all it has to offer.

Look at the small things you can change to build the life you deserve to live. Think about how you spend your first moments of the day. Listen to how you talk to yourself. Take control of what you consume. Recognize who you surround yourself with every day. Acknowledge how you respond to mistakes and setbacks.

These are the small, yet hugely significant things you can control, once you know how. In my experience, if you get a handle on the little things, it can make the big things less daunting. Remember, how you live each day is how you live your life. In fact, the little things generally turn out to be the big things.

As I enter the next phase of my life – motherhood – I am filled with so many emotions. I could let them overwhelm me, but I choose to take control and be confident in my capabilities. I know life, and my experiences so far, have taught me the skills and coping mechanisms to be the best version of myself as I adapt to this new role. I will fail. I will fall. But I'll get back up again and keep going.

And this is the thing – life is a continuum, it is constantly in flux, and we are presented with the most unexpected things at the most random of times. If we approach life with a sense of purpose, of positivity, with the knowledge that we might not always get it right, then we will do our very best in the process. We are all learning, just make sure that you are living, otherwise all the learning will go to waste. It all starts with having the courage to try.

You can do tough things! Go do them!

Acknowledgements

I actually struggled with this section of the book because, in truth, there are so many people I would like to acknowledge, but it would be like doing the Leaving Cert exams all over again – I'd have to put my hand up and ask for 'additional paper'. The reason being, if I started to list all the people who inspired and/ or supported me along the way we'd be here a while, so I'll try to keep this brief (there's a first for everything, eh!).

Thank you to Michael McLoughlin and the team at Penguin Random House Ireland for all of the Trojan work you put into making this book a reality.

Special thanks to the brilliant Patricia Deevy for your endless advice, support – and patience – throughout the process. Thank you for sharing my enthusiasm for the vision of this book from the outset, and for all the interesting and insightful conversations in which we fleshed out what the book could look like.

To Claire Pelly, my wonderful and talented editor. Thank you for all the late-night exchanges and endless voice notes. Thank you for 'getting me' and understanding the essence of what I wanted this book to be. You helped to take my words and ideas to a new level, a level I couldn't have achieved on my own. You turned this book into something I'm so proud of. You went above and beyond, and it was truly appreciated.

ACKNOWLEDGEMENTS

We all need people in our corner. To those in my corner – you know who you are – I am so grateful to have you in my life. In particular, a shout-out to my pals Claire and Bríd. Claire, thank you for meeting with me in that coffee shop in Blanchardstown, back when this book was just swirling around in my head. You were one of the first people I spoke to about this project as I knew, my wise friend, that you would be a wealth of knowledge. Bríd, thank you for being a true friend, for lifting me up during this writing process, for reminding me I was capable. You did this without even realizing it. Real queens fix each other's crowns. You are a true queen!

To the Niamhs at NK Management – thank you for brainstorming with me in the early days. Niamh T, thank you for giving me the encouragement – and the gentle nudge – I needed to write this book. Thank you for the ongoing belief and support.

To the voice in my head that at times told me 'I couldn't'. Overcoming that voice has been key to growing my resilience and stepping out of my comfort zone again and again. We can all tell ourselves we can't. But we usually can! We can try new things, change jobs, move countries, set up new businesses, write books. WE. CAN. DO. TOUGH. THINGS. But the first and most crucial step is pushing past the internal voice that tells us we shouldn't give it a go.

To Mam, thank you for always being on the other end of the phone, for allowing me to vent and ramble. Thank you for our numerous chats about everything and anything to take my mind off my 'writer's block' whenever it hit. And thank you for always listening. I'm lucky to have you.

To Dad, thank you for my competitive instinct and (stubborn) determination. Let's face it, you probably wouldn't have read this book, but you would have immensely enjoyed others quoting snippets of it to you. And you would have been proud that I had the courage to put pen to paper. It's hard to write these words in the past tense, but I know you are still with me.

To Ronan, thank you for uncovering a new depth of love, strength and vulnerability within me. I want to be the best person and mum I can be for you. Be patient with me, though, I'm learning on the job.

To Kev, thank you for being my first editor. Thank you for being my sounding board on our many walks and for being my pep-talk giver. Thank you for the countless times – even in the dead of night – that you reassured me, when I was nervous about sharing stories I've never shared before. I trust you wholeheartedly to always have my back.

And finally, to you, the readers, thank you for picking up my book (providing you don't put it back down on the shelf!). Thank you for giving me your time, as it's your most valuable asset. My hope is that by reading this book, it will help you to realize that you are brilliant and truly deserving of the life you want. Go get it!